Quality Control in the Assisted Reproductive Technology Laboratory

This book provides an overview of quality control in ART laboratories. It explores frameworks and essential tools necessary for effective quality management. The fields of monitoring, equipment maintenance, and the intricate aspects of embryo care and cryopreservation are thoroughly examined. The significance of the ART lab witnessing system is highlighted, demonstrating the seamless integration of both manual and electronic witnessing tools. Readers will gain insights into the roles played by KPIs and SOPs. For aspiring embryologists, this guide offers an exploration of training techniques, addressing the inherent challenges of the field. Practical coping strategies are provided to help navigate these stressors successfully.

With real-world case studies and discussions on laboratory design, this resource serves as a guide to achieving excellence in ART. It emphasises the importance of balancing patient care, procedural accuracy, and practitioner well-being.

Durai P is Senior Embryologist at KIMS Hospital Hyderabad, India.

Reproductive Medicine and Assisted Reproductive Techniques Series

About the Series

The world of reproductive medicine has grown greatly in size and complexity since the first IVF baby was born. The *Reproductive Medicine & Assisted Reproductive Techniques* series keeps readers up to date with the latest laboratory and clinical techniques for improving successful birth rates. Each volume in the series is prepared independently and typically focuses on a topical theme. Volumes are published on an occasional basis, according to the emergence of noteworthy scientific developments.

For more information about this series please visit: www.routledge.com/Reproductive-Medicine-and-Assisted-Reproductive-Techniques-Series/book-series/IHCRMEDASREP

Quality Control in the Assisted Reproductive Technology Laboratory

Durai P
Head, Embryology Lab Services
Department of Reproductive Medicine
Krishna Institute of Medical Sciences (KIMS Hospital)
Hyderabad, India

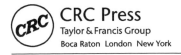

CRC Press
Taylor & Francis Group
Boca Raton London New York

CRC Press is an imprint of the
Taylor & Francis Group, an **informa** business

Designed cover image: Shutterstock

First edition published 2024
by CRC Press
2385 NW Executive Center Drive, Suite 320, Boca Raton FL 33431

and by CRC Press
4 Park Square, Milton Park, Abingdon, Oxon, OX14 4RN

CRC Press is an imprint of Taylor & Francis Group, LLC

© 2024 Durai P

ISBN: 978-1-032-62272-9 (hbk)
ISBN: 978-1-032-62026-8 (pbk)
ISBN: 978-1-032-62273-6 (ebk)

DOI: 10.1201/9781032622736

Typeset in Palatino LT Std
by Apex CoVantage, LLC

Dedicated to patients who are bravely facing the challenges of infertility,

and to all the embryologists and clinicians who work

tirelessly to make patients' dreams come true.

Contents

Preface

The rapidly evolving field of assisted reproductive technology (ART) has been a beacon of hope and possibilities for countless couples struggling with infertility. The history of ART dates back to the birth of the first "test-tube baby," Louise Brown, in 1978, marking a milestone in the successful application of in vitro fertilisation (IVF). Since then, ART has undergone significant advancements, encompassing a range of techniques. As ART labs continue to innovate, maintaining high-quality standards and adhering to best practices becomes increasingly crucial.

Quality Control in Assisted Reproductive Technology Labs is a comprehensive guide designed to provide embryologists, clinicians, lab technicians, and other stakeholders with an in-depth understanding of the quality control measures required in IVF labs and practical guidance on their effective implementation.

Drawing on real-life case studies, examples of logs and SOPs, and lessons learned from mishaps in IVF labs around the world, this book highlights the importance of quality control and offers practical insights and strategies for enhancing the efficiency and overall performance of ART labs. By focusing on both the technical and human aspects of quality control, this guide aims to equip readers with the knowledge and tools needed to consistently deliver the highest standard of care.

The guide provides insights into the complex regulatory compliance landscape, with an overview of ART lab regulations from various countries. The diversity of legal frameworks and the challenges faced by professionals working in different regulatory environments are clearly laid out.

The content herein has been carefully curated to empower professionals in the ART field to provide exceptional care to their patients, continuously improve their practices, and drive the field of assisted reproduction forward.

In conclusion, I express my deepest gratitude to everyone who contributed to this project. My profound thanks go to Dr S Vyjayanthi for her instrumental guidance and Dr M. Prasad for generously sharing his scientific insights. I would like to extend my appreciation to the management of KIMS Hospital for their unwavering support. I sincerely thank Robert Peden, the commissioning editor, for his guidance throughout this journey.

I am grateful to my family for their support and encouragement. I also wish to acknowledge the resilience of all professionals and patients in the ART field, whose experiences have greatly enriched this book. Finally, thanks to the entire editorial and production team for their attention to detail, ensuring a high-quality final product.

This book is a testament to the power of collective knowledge and the relentless pursuit of excellence in the field of ART. As we move forward, I hope this resource serves as an essential tool, contributing to this field's continued success and evolution.

1

Introduction to QC in ART Labs

There are three principles in the field of assisted reproductive technology (ART), quality control (QC), quality assurance (QA), and good laboratory practices (GLPs), that serve as the pillars of laboratory operation. The foremost objective of QC is to ensure that laboratory processes and outcomes meet quality standards; this entails monitoring the performance of equipment, handling samples, and thorough testing of products to identify and resolve any potential issues.

On the other hand, QA focuses on maintaining the high quality benchmarks established by QC methods. Key components of QA include developing and implementing standard operating procedures (SOPs), conducting external audits, and regularly evaluating laboratory procedures to identify areas for improvement.

GLPs constitute a framework to ensure the reliability, repeatability, and accuracy of laboratory results. This is achieved through training of personnel, recording of data, and diligent maintenance of equipment. The synergy between QC, QA, and GLP creates a system that enhances accuracy in ART laboratories, strengthening the validation of results.

To ensure the integration of QC, QA, and GLP in ART facilities, it is essential to have defined goals and measurable standards for evaluating performance. The implementation of key performance indicators (KPIs) plays a role in achieving this. By monitoring and assessing KPIs, ART laboratories can pinpoint any issues and take the necessary actions to improve the effectiveness of their processes.

The interplay between QC, QA, and GLP within ART laboratories is crucial for maintaining a quality management system. QC primarily concentrates on monitoring equipment performance and managing sample handling processes to ensure consistency across parameters. Whenever any inconsistencies are detected, QA measures such as audits come into play, facilitating corrective actions to rectify the issues.

Standard operating procedures are the outcome of QA efforts and play a role in bringing uniformity to laboratory procedures. By establishing protocols, SOPs directly contribute to the accuracy and reproducibility of lab results.

GLP specifically emphasises personnel training, ensuring that laboratory staff possess the required skills for their designated roles. Moreover, GLP principles advocate for data documentation and practical storage systems, which ultimately promote accurate results recording.

In the context of ART laboratories, QC serves as an approach to inspecting and monitoring laboratory processes. Its primary objective is to achieve predictable results while minimising errors. The ultimate goal of QC in ART labs is to optimise the success rate of ART techniques and to enhance care. Any inconsistencies or deviations can have consequences for treatment outcomes, impacting the emotional and financial well-being of patients.

Internal quality control (IQC) and external quality control (EQC) play roles in monitoring and assessing laboratory processes. For example, environmental monitoring in ART labs involves checks on air quality, water quality, and surfaces to identify contaminants. Additionally, regular calibration of equipments, assessment of media quality evaluations of personnel competency, and quality control testing are components of QC in ART labs.

DOI: 10.1201/9781032622736-1

1.1 Schematic Overview

To effectively understand and implement quality measures in an in vitro fertilisation (IVF) laboratory, it is essential to have a comprehensive understanding of the IVF lab process to help identify points and areas where errors may occur during operations.

This schematic approach does not assist in problem-solving; instead, it highlights areas that may require more attention or improvement. By providing a framework for examining the IVF process, it ensures that every step in the process is carefully considered and all possible concerns are adequately addressed (Figure 1.1).

The Role of QC: ART procedures such as in vito fertilisation (IVF), intracytoplasmic sperm injection (ICSI), and preimplantation genetic testing (PGT) are intricate and costly. Hence, a comprehensive QC programme is indispensable for ensuring safety and optimising treatment effectiveness. The key roles of QC in ART labs include safeguarding well-being, enhancing ART outcomes, adhering to regulations and standards, and providing reassurance to patients.

The importance of QC: The significance of QC in ART labs cannot be emphasised enough. Its contribution to achieving ART outcomes is paramount. QC monitors and documents physical and chemical parameters such as culture media to ensure the accuracy of equipment and enable prompt maintenance when necessary. Furthermore, QC plays a role in maintaining laboratory conditions, handling andrology procedures, conducting embryo culture, and selecting embryos for transfer. Adhering to procedure protocols is vital to ART procedures such as IVF and ICSI, where even minor deviations can have a substantial impact on success rates.

The implementation of total quality management systems (TQM) plays a role in an ART lab. TQMS embody an approach that prioritises quality and continuous improvement,

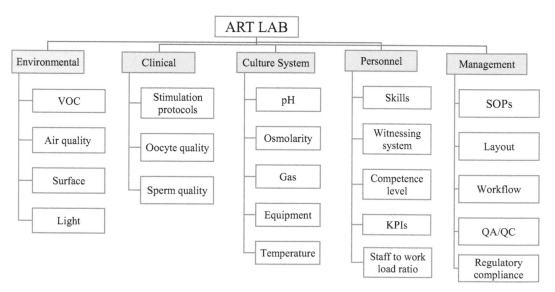

FIGURE 1.1
Schematic overview of ART lab.

involving all levels of the organisation. Within the realm of embryology, TQMS aim to optimise processes from oocyte retrieval to embryo transfer or freezing. This approach emphasises high quality standards, ultimately elevating the success rate of IVF procedures and enhancing satisfaction. Integrating TQMS within ART labs is not merely a luxury—it is an imperative. It guarantees the provision of high-quality services to patients, augmenting the likelihood of positive outcomes and upholding the long-term viability of lab operations.

1.2 Regulatory Overview: ART Labs and Embryologists Worldwide

The field of ART continuously offers advanced solutions to couples facing fertility challenges. However, it also raises social and ethical considerations that require careful examination. Key concerns revolve around the misuse or abuse of this technology, limited accessibility due to costs, and the safety implications for both individuals undergoing ART procedures and the children conceived through these methods.

The high expenses associated with ART procedures can lead to limited access to treatment, exacerbating the socioeconomic divide by creating disparities between those who can afford these advanced reproductive treatments and those who cannot. Consequently, the opportunity to conceive children with the help of ART is unevenly distributed among individuals. Furthermore, safety is a concern within the realm of ART, as it encompasses risks such as the occurrence of multiple pregnancies, premature births, and potential long-term health effects on the children conceived through ART.

Non-medical applications of ART, like gender selection or the prospect of creating 'designer babies', are topics of ongoing debate. The underlying concern arises from the possibility of prioritising certain traits over others, a shift that could fundamentally alter societal values and expectations.

It is crucial for the industry to prioritise enhancing the accessibility and affordability of ART while also preventing its medical misuse. When using donor gametes or embryos, it is important to handle considerations like informed consent, privacy protection, and the well-being of individuals who are conceived through donor-assisted procedures with care.

To address these concerns, regulatory agencies and professional organisations have set up guidelines for ART labs. While specific requirements may vary across regions, the overall commitment to maintaining practices and delivering top-quality care remains consistent across the board.

1.3 ART Regulations in the United States of America

The responsibility of overseeing ART in the United States of America (USA) primarily falls on the Food and Drug Administration (FDA). The FDA's role involves monitoring the handling of donor eggs, sperm, and embryos across ART labs and fertility clinics. The FDA's strict protocols aim to guarantee safe treatments. Non-compliance with these standards can lead to fines, licence suspensions, or other penalties, emphasising the FDA's role in upholding the integrity of ART practices.

In addition to the FDA, the Centers for Disease Control and Prevention (CDC) also plays a part in regulating ART in the United States. The CDC reports data related to ART practices nationwide through the National Assisted Reproductive Surveillance System (NASS). This comprehensive data allows the CDC to closely monitor and evaluate ART outcomes. The reports furnish insights into success rates, birth occurrences, and other important statistics. This robust evidence base enables evaluation of the safety and effectiveness of ART procedures. The Society for Assisted Reproductive Technology (SART) is another organisation involved in regulating ART within the community. SART upholds clinical standards by providing guidance to ART clinics and laboratories, thereby ensuring excellence in their practices.

Some places require insurance companies to include ART procedures in their coverage to guarantee that people can receive the treatments they need. Additionally, certain states have put regulations in place to ensure the safety of patients and donors when using donor eggs, embryos, and surrogates. However, the fact that regulations vary from state to state emphasises the need for policies that address insurance coverage for ART.

1.3.1 For Embryologists

In the United States, individuals aspiring to become embryologists typically pursue a bachelor's degree in biology or a related field as a foundation for acquiring the knowledge required for this profession. Specialised training in embryology further hones their skills and expertise. Professional bodies such as the American Board of Bioanalysis (ABB) and the American Association of Bioanalysts (AAB) offer certification programmes to enhance professionalism within the field.

However, regulatory standards for embryologists vary throughout the country, leading to disparities. For instance, states such as New York and Florida mandate that embryologists obtain a licence in order to practice, underscoring the need for regulations that ensure embryologists meet established qualifications and adhere to safety-focused guidelines.

1.4 ART Regulations in Brazil

In Brazil, there is a body called the Federal Council of Medicine (CFM) that provides guidelines for aspects of ART. These guidelines were initially established in 1992 and have been regularly updated to keep up with advances in technology. Clinics offering ART services in Brazil are required to obtain accreditation from the CFM, and it is mandatory for these clinics to adhere to the provided guidelines.

Embryologists in Brazil typically hold degrees in the sciences or medicine and then receive specialised training in embryology or human reproduction. To become certified embryologists, they must meet the requirements set out by the Brazilian Society of Assisted Reproduction (SBRA) or other professional organisations.

1.5 ART Regulations in Europe

Each country in Europe has its own set of rules and regulations for ART; this approach allows countries to adapt their regulations to fit local legal and ethical considerations.

By adopting country-specific regulations, European nations can address the perspectives and values within their societies, ensuring that ART practices are conducted in a way that respects and reflects the context of each nation.

In addition to regulations, pan-European organisations play a role in creating detailed guidelines and recommendations for ART facilities. These organisations are crucial in establishing and promoting procedures and best practices across Europe. They formulate guidelines that ensure the quality, safety, and ethical implementation of ART procedures. They also provide educational programmes and credentials for professionals in the field. Renowned institutions including the European Society of Human Reproduction and Embryology (ESHRE) and the European IVF Monitoring Consortium (EIM) contribute knowledge. It is crucial for ART clinics and practitioners to stay up to date on regulations in their countries to ensure compliance and provide safe and ethical ART services.

In the European Union, there are regulations governing the use of tissues and gametes in ART. The EU's Directive on Tissues and Cells (Directive 2004/23/EC) mandates that ART labs adhere to good manufacturing practices (GMPs) and GLPs. They are also required to maintain records and report any events. Additionally, the European Union stipulates that ART laboratories must comply with ISO 15189, which is a recognised standard for medical laboratories.

Furthermore, there are guidelines provided by organisations such as the European Society of Human Reproduction and Embryology. ESHRE is a body comprising ART clinics and practitioners offering guidance and recommendations for ART clinics and laboratories. It provides directives in areas such as donor gametes, preimplantation genetic testing, and managing stimulation in IVF cycles. It is worth noting that individual countries may have their own guidelines or regulations pertaining to ART practices alongside those provided by ESHRE.

1.6 ART Regulations in France

In France, the French Biomedicine Agency is responsible for overseeing the rules and regulations surrounding ART. They ensure that ART is implemented in accordance with the French Bioethics Law, which establishes guidelines for the use of gametes and embryos. To comply with these regulations, the agency sets standards for ART practitioners, including their training and certification. Quality control measures are also in place to monitor and report on ART procedures and their outcomes. It is worth noting that in France, gamete donations are kept anonymous, and donors are not allowed to make contact with their offspring.

In France, professionals working in the field of embryology usually hold a university degree in the sciences or a related field. Additionally, they undergo specialised training specifically focused on embryology, ensuring that they meet the laboratory standards set in the country.

1.7 ART Regulations in Spain

The Spanish Fertility Society (SEF) is responsible for formulating guidelines for ART applications in Spain.

In Spain, embryologists commonly have a background in biology, medicine, pharmacy, biochemistry, or biotechnology. They also undergo training in reproduction to become experts in this field. Additionally, they have the opportunity to obtain certification through the Spanish Association for the Study of Biology and Reproduction (Asociación para el Estudio de la Biología de la Reproducción; ASEBIR) to reflect their level of professional competence.

1.7.1 For Embryologists

In the United Kingdom, embryologists who work in ART clinics are required to register with the Human Fertilisation and Embryology Authority (HFEA), which serves as the body overseeing ART implementation. These embryologists follow the HFEA Code of Practice, which provides guidelines and standards to ensure quality control and optimal patient care in ART procedures. Typically, embryologists have specialised education and training in embryology. Many also hold a certificate from or are registered with the Association of Clinical Embryologists (ACE).

In Europe, embryologists are expected to have a degree in biology or a related field. ESHRE encourages professionals in the field to enhance their expertise by pursuing certifications. One such certification programme offered by ESHRE is the Certification for Clinical Embryologists (CCE). The CCE programme involves education and training followed by an examination, and it is recognised throughout Europe. This certification validates the competency of individuals working as embryologists. Moreover, ESHRE provides training opportunities to support the growth of embryologists and keep them updated with advancements in reproductive medicine.

1.8 ART Regulations in Australia

In Australia, the National Health and Medical Research Council (NHMRC), a government organisation, closely oversees the application of ART. The council plays a role in providing guidance, funding, and nationwide support for health and medical research.

To operate in Australia, ART clinics must obtain a licence from the Reproductive Technology Accreditation Committee (RTAC) and abide by the standards outlined in the NHMRC's Ethical Guidelines. These guidelines govern the use of ART in both practice and research. Specific regulations are in place regarding the use of donor gametes; these determine how many families a single donor can contribute to and allow donors to set conditions for their gametes' usage. Additionally, individuals conceived through donor gametes have the right to access identifying information about their donors once they reach adulthood.

Regarding surrogacy, Australia permits only those arrangements in which the surrogate receives compensation solely for expenses incurred. Before entering into such an arrangement, both the intended parents and the surrogate must undergo counselling.

ART clinics in Australia have an obligation to report data, including success rates, incidents, and other outcomes, to the Australian and New Zealand Assisted Reproduction Database (ANZARD).

1.8.1 For Embryologists

For those aspiring to be embryologists, it is important to know that embryologists and ART laboratories in Australia adhere to the guidelines of the National Health and Medical

Research Council and the Reproductive Technology Accreditation Committee. To pursue a career in embryology, individuals must hold qualifications in embryology, biotechnology, or a related life science field. Furthermore, they are required to undergo training in embryology, and they may need accreditation from organisations like the Fertility Society of Australia (FSA) or the Australian Association of Clinical Embryologists (AACE).

1.9 ART Regulations in China

The Chinese government has implemented regulations for ART due to the country's population and the challenges associated with infertility. The Ministry of Health and the National Health and Family Planning Commission are responsible for overseeing the practice of ART in China.

To operate in China, ART clinics are required to obtain a licence from the National Health Commission of the People's Republic of China. These clinics must also adhere to the standards and guidelines established by the Chinese Medical Association.

The qualifications for embryologists in China are rigorous. Typically, they are required to hold a degree in life sciences, biotechnology, or clinical embryology. Additionally, they must undergo training in embryology. They must obtain certification from the Chinese Society for Reproductive Medicine or a similar professional organisation.

1.10 ART Regulations in Japan

In Japan, the Japan Society of Obstetrics and Gynaecology (JSOG) plays a role in overseeing assisted technologies like in vitro fertilisation. This organisation establishes guidelines and regulations that clinics and practitioners must follow.

For clinics in Japan that provide ART services, it is necessary to obtain licences and accreditations from the Ministry of Health, Labour, and Welfare. These clinics are obligated to adhere to the guidelines provided by JSOG, which are also mandated by the government. Embryologists in Japan typically have a background in life sciences or medicine and undergo further training in embryology. Certification from JSOG or a similar professional organisation is often a requirement.

1.11 ART Regulations in India

In 2020 India introduced the ART Regulation Bill with the aim of governing ART procedures and the practice of surrogacy. This proposed legislation seeks to establish state boards that will ensure compliance with ART regulations. These boards will oversee ART practices across the country and focus on regulating ART within states.

Under the law, all ART clinics and practitioners are required to register with the national board and undergo inspections to guarantee they meet the standards. The legislation also provides guidelines for the storage and disposal of gametes and embryos, as well as limiting the number of embryos that can be transferred during IVF treatments. Furthermore, it allows surrogacy for couples who face challenges with conception while strictly prohibiting any form of surrogacy that could lead to exploitation or harm to the women involved.

Furthermore, the ART bill proposes the establishment of a registry and accreditation authority for overseeing ART clinics and banks across the country. Per this law, the regulatory authority is obligated to create and manage a database that includes all ART clinics and banks operating throughout India. This law sets forth rules and regulations for conducting ART procedures in India. The primary objectives are to prioritise the safety and efficiency of these procedures while safeguarding the welfare and rights of both patients and donors engaged in these practices.

In compliance with the legislation governing ART and surrogacy, practitioners in this field must fulfil training criteria. They should hold a degree in embryology, biotechnology, or life sciences. They must also receive training related to ART procedures at clinics that adhere to Level 2 standards; this ensures that these professionals possess the expertise and capabilities to carry out ART procedures with safety and effectiveness.

1.12 The Impact of the ART Bill 2020

The ART Bill 2020 aims to enhance care and minimise risks associated with assisted technologies. A key aspect of this bill is the creation of a database for ART clinics, which ensures consistency in practices and safeguards patient rights.

Quality assurance measures: The bill brings about advancements in the regulation of ART clinics. It sets out requirements that ART clinics must adhere to, such as employing healthcare professionals like medical practitioners, embryologists, and counsellors. Additionally, it emphasises the need for facilities and adherence to safety protocols. By implementing quality assurance checks, ART clinics strive to improve the reliability, accuracy, and safety of their procedures. These measures include monitoring the environment, calibrating equipment, and following maintenance protocols to uphold the standards of ART practices.

Record-keeping obligations: Another important provision in the bill is the requirement for ART clinics to maintain records for a minimum of 10 years. This ensures accountability and transparency, allowing for the traceability of procedures. The bill gives the national authority the ability to inspect these records to ensure compliance and quality control, ultimately safeguarding the rights of patients and donors.

Enhanced accountability for ART clinics: The new legislation places an emphasis on accountability by establishing a board for ART clinics. This regulatory body will oversee the implementation of the law and evaluate the operations of ART clinics nationwide. Its purpose is to promote accountability and ensure that clinics comply with the standards, thus leading to improved patient outcomes.

Patients' rights: One crucial aspect of this bill is the protection of patients' rights. It guarantees that patients have access to counselling services, where they receive information about the outcomes and risks associated with the procedures. The bill also necessitates consent, ensuring that individuals fully comprehend the implications of the treatments before making a decision. Additionally, it establishes a framework to safeguard the rights and wellbeing of children born through ART procedures.

By encouraging clinics to adhere to regulations, this bill works towards instilling trust in the safety and effectiveness of ART procedures. With a focus on transparency and accountability, the ART Bill 2020 creates an environment where patients feel more assured about the quality of services they receive.

CHAPTER 1

SUMMARY

- Implementing quality control is integral to the operations of assisted reproductive technology laboratories, ensuring the reliability and precision of equipment, processes, and personnel. This commitment to QC helps identify and address potential issues as early as possible, thereby enhancing the overall success rate of ART procedures.

- The emphasis on QC measures contributes to improved treatment outcomes by maintaining stringent standards across all stages of the ART process. It facilitates the execution of each step accurately and efficiently, thus significantly improving success rates.

- A robust QC system is instrumental in building and maintaining patient trust. It guarantees the quality and safety of ART procedures, fostering confidence in the treatments provided.

- Compliance with QC protocols is a key determinant of the regulatory adherence of ART labs. This adherence varies with the jurisdiction and ensures that the labs operate within the bounds of the law.

- QC processes also foster a culture of continuous improvement, with ongoing evaluation and refinement of ART lab practices. This culture of improvement enhances the overall quality of ART procedures and contributes to advancements in patient care.

- Total quality management systems (TQMSs) are indispensable to ART labs, bolstering their quality and success rates. The focus of TQMS on continuous improvement, proficiency testing, and environmental monitoring creates a collaborative atmosphere conducive to the maintenance of high standards.

- The regulatory oversight of ART labs varies on a global scale, reflecting the diverse contexts within which these laboratories operate. The United States observes regulations from the CDC, SART, and CLIA and guidelines from the American Society for Reproductive Medicine (ASRM), while Europe follows guidelines and best practices developed by ESHRE. China's ART labs are governed by the NHC's guidelines, which emphasise personnel qualifications, laboratory conditions, equipment, and quality management systems.

- Australia's ART labs operate under the guidelines established by the FSA and RTAC, focusing on personnel qualifications, laboratory conditions, equipment, and the quality management system. They require proper accreditation for labs to operate.

- Regulatory compliance is paramount for ART labs. It ensures the maintenance of quality and safety standards in assisted reproductive procedures, minimises risks, improves patient outcomes, and fortifies trust among patients and the community.

- The process of regular inspections and evaluations is crucial to upholding high standards in ART labs, promoting a culture of transparency and accountability.

- Despite the differences in regulations for QC in ART labs across the world, the ultimate objective remains universal: to achieve and maintain the highest possible standards in ART procedures. This objective centres on promoting successful outcomes.

2

Internal Quality Control and External Quality Control

2.1 Control Samples

Control samples play a role in evaluating the accuracy and dependability of test results. They help ensure that the outcomes are in line with expectations and serve as a way to identify any inconsistencies or positive indications.

To maintain consistency, laboratories establish acceptance criteria that define the expected range for control sample outcomes. These samples are evaluated using the same methodologies. If the observed results deviate from the predetermined range, steps should be taken to investigate and address any anomalies.

When it comes to control samples, readily available products are often preferred due to their user-friendly nature and traceability to reference standards. They enable monitoring of semen test precision in terms of count, motility, and morphology.

Alternatively, laboratories can also recommend using in-house–prepared controls. These customised control samples can be tailored to testing situations and may prove cost effective as well as meeting sample requirements.

Choosing control samples that accurately represent the expected values of the tested samples is crucial. To ensure accurate results, it is recommended to test the control samples on the same equipment as the actual samples.

2.2 Frequency of Internal QC

The complexity of a test can impact the frequency of internal quality control checks.

Test volume:

With the increasing number of tests conducted, the likelihood of encountering inconsistencies may also grow. It is essential to assess and oversee quality control to promptly detect and correct any variations that may arise during the testing procedure; this ensures that the test outcomes remain accurate and dependable.

Historical performance: The frequency of conducting internal quality control may be influenced by the performance of the facility. If there have been cases where

DOI: 10.1201/9781032622736-2

unreliable results were produced, it may be advisable to increase the frequency of QC; this will ensure that any issues are detected and addressed promptly.

Data analysis: During data analysis, the outcomes of control measures are compared to predetermined limits or target values. Any patterns or trends that could potentially signal an issue are carefully examined.

Levey-Jennings charts: These charts are frequently utilised to evaluate internal quality control results. Control boundaries are determined using real-life data, and any observations outside of these boundaries are regarded as deviations.

Statistical analysis: The process of statistical analysis applies specific methods to IQC data with the objective of identifying patterns that could indicate potential errors. One approach is to use regression analysis to examine changes in control data over a given timeframe. Another method involves utilising ANOVA to compare control samples and detect any variations.

2.3 External Quality Control

Taking part in quality control activities like proficiency testing programmes and comparisons between laboratories helps ensure that labs maintain the highest possible level of quality in their processes, equipment, and staff performance.

2.4 Proficiency Testing Programmes

- The initial step in the programme involves registration and enrolment. Laboratories are mandated to supply information regarding their capabilities and specify the tests for which they need to undergo proficiency testing.

- The proficiency testing provider supplies samples that mimic real-life specimens. These samples are designed to imitate cases and are typically provided without any knowledge of the expected results.

- Personnel who participate in the programme analyse these samples using their established methods and submit their findings to the proficiency testing provider before a given deadline.

- During the evaluation phase, the proficiency testing provider compares the results with expected outcomes, assessing accuracy, precision, and correctness.

- Once the evaluation is complete, all participants receive a report from the proficiency testing provider, which offers feedback on their performance. The report highlights both strengths and areas that need improvement. If any issues are identified in the feedback, it is essential for labs to promptly address them by taking action.

Consistently participating in proficiency testing programmes is highly recommended for labs, as it helps maintain accreditation and demonstrates a commitment to quality assurance.

2.5 Inter-Laboratory Comparisons

Through the systematic analysis of experimental methodologies and the evaluation of corresponding outcomes, significant insights can be acquired, contributing to the continuous improvement of protocols.

> **Sample exchange:** This method involves sharing and examining samples using their respective testing procedures. The outcomes are subsequently compared to evaluate the reliability and precision of the techniques employed in each lab.

The steps involved in a sample exchange process are listed in the following.

- **Selections:** The selection process involves choosing laboratories that possess the required testing capabilities and interests to participate in the sample exchange exercises.
- **Preparation and distribution:** Each lab dispatches samples to the collaborating testing facilities.
- **Analysis of samples:** The laboratories analyse the samples they receive, adhering to their SOPs.
- **Discussion and feedback:** The research facilities participating in the study maintain communication with each other. They share data, discuss their observations, and offer feedback to improve their testing methods.

These steps help maintain a high-quality approach to testing by ensuring the participants in the sample exchange exercise follow procedures.

2.6 Exchange of Personnel

Embryologists or technicians from one laboratory frequently partake in visits to observe and evaluate the methodologies utilised by their colleagues in a different testing facility.

2.7 Steps in Personnel Exchange

- Identifying partners: Laboratories with similar interests and goals are selected for the exchange programme.

- Planning and scheduling visits: Visits are strategically coordinated and arranged based on the mutual availability and convenience of the laboratories involved in accordance with established protocols.
- Observations and evaluations: Visiting personnel observe and evaluate the host test centre's practices, focusing on sample handling, testing protocols, and data analysis.
- Sharing of knowledge and expertise: Both parties share their experiences, insights, and best practices to help improve each other's performance.
- Follow-up: The process of follow-up and continuous improvement involves implementing the best practices and continually monitoring their performance for ongoing enhancements.

2.8 Collaborative Research Projects

ART labs frequently participate in collaborative research endeavours, undertaking the evaluation of methodologies and achievements. This activity enhances the lab personnel's understanding of the factors influencing ART outcomes. Such collaboration allows for the acquisition of valuable insights and the development of standardised protocols, ultimately providing benefits to the entire field.

2.9 Steps Involved in Research Projects

- Selecting research topics: The process of selecting research topics in the lab involves identifying subjects that align with the interests and areas of expertise within the laboratory team.
- Forming research teams: Researchers come together and form teams to work on the chosen research topic.
- Developing study protocols: The research teams collaborate to create methods for data collection, ensuring consistency across the study.
- Conducting the study: Each participant carries out the study according to the agreed protocols for collecting data.
- Publishing results: The research findings are shared among the scientific community through publication in peer-reviewed scientific journals and presentations at conferences.

2.10 Addressing Discrepancies

ART laboratories should take immediate action to address any discrepancies in external quality control effects or feedback that highlights areas for improvement.

2.10.1 Review Testing Protocols

- Evaluating sample handling and preparation techniques
- Assessing the efficacy and calibration of equipment
- Examining the data analysis and interpretation methods
- Verifying the consistency of laboratory practices

2.10.2 Comparison of Methods with Other Centres

- Engaging in inter-comparison and proficiency testing programmes
- Consulting with experts in the field to gain insights into best practices

2.10.3 Corrective Actions

- Modifying testing protocols to eliminate any potential sources of error
- Upgrading or recalibrating equipment as needed
- Providing additional training to staff to improve their skills and understanding of the testing processes
- Implementing quality control measures to prevent future discrepancies

2.10.4 Re-Evaluation of Performance

- Participating in additional rounds of proficiency testing or inter-comparisons
- Conducting regular audits of practices

2.11 Analytical QC in ART Laboratory Tests

2.11.1 Sperm Count

Routine sperm analysis assessments are performed as part of fertility testing services. The accuracy and precision of sperm analysis reports greatly depend on maintaining quality control measures. These measures are crucial for maintaining and improving the success of ART treatments.

To ensure the accuracy and precision of these assessments that follow analytical QC measures, the following steps are taken.

Using control samples: In addition to collecting samples, the testing facility utilises control samples containing known concentrations of sperm to validate its method of sperm counting.

Checking counting chamber quality: Personnel carefully inspect chambers for scratches, debris, and other defects that could affect the counting process. Any chambers that do not meet quality standards are replaced.

These techniques can improve the accuracy of sperm count measurements and contribute to the observed results in patients undergoing ART treatments.

Monitoring and documenting the outcomes of QC indicators: Facilities diligently maintain comprehensive records of control sample data, calibration records, and staff training activities.

Assessing embryos: For embryo assessment, it is crucial to use precise techniques to ensure the highest standards of quality in the evaluation process.

- ART labs utilise scoring systems, such as the Gardner and Schoolcraft system, to evaluate embryo morphology. These systems assign numerical scores to embryos based on their specific characteristics.

- **External quality assessment schemes:** Labs actively engage in multiple external quality assessment schemes to ensure the highest standards and compare their performance to industry benchmarks. These methodologies encompass proficiency testing initiatives, inter-laboratory comparisons, and the process of accreditation.

- **Internal quality control:** To ensure the reliability of embryo assessments, IQC procedures are employed. The processes encompass the verification of embryonic scores to monitor the efficacy of various assessment techniques as well as periodic evaluations of the assessment protocols.

2.12 Process of Troubleshooting in the ART Lab

Procedures encompass a series of systematic actions and cautious manipulation of materials. It is imperative to employ efficient problem-solving techniques to prioritise the well-being of patients, enhance the rates of successful treatment, and uphold one's reputation. This process entails the identification, diagnosis, and resolution of any potential issues that may occur during various stages of ART (Figure 2.1).

2.13 Identifying the Issue

- Be familiar with SOPs and expected outcomes for oocyte retrieval, sperm preparation, fertilisation, embryo culture, and embryo transfer.

- Stay vigilant for unexpected or unusual values that may indicate issues within the lab's practices. These could include poor fertilisation rates, embryo arrest, or low implantation rates.

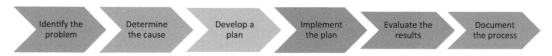

FIGURE 2.1
Steps in ART lab troubleshooting.

2.14 Gathering Information

- Review the records of the procedures performed to check if there were any deviations from the SOPs that might explain the issue.
- Check the logs of the equipment used to see if there were any maintenance, calibration, or usage problems that could have contributed to the problem.
- Assess the quality and expiration dates of the reagents used in the procedures, since compromised reagents can affect the outcomes.
- Take into consideration factors like temperature, humidity, and air quality, as they can influence ART techniques and their outcomes.
- Organise patient demographics and outcomes to thoroughly analyse the issue.
- Analyse all the collected information to identify the root cause(s) of the problem.

2.15 Consulting Resources

- Scientific literature: To understand the identified problem, it is advisable to conduct an examination of pertinent research papers, case studies, and protocols to explore its potential origins.
- Optimal methodologies for the industry: When confronted with particular challenges, it is recommended to consult authoritative guidelines from reputable organisations such as the ESHRE or the ASRM.
- Engaging in discussions through forums and communities of experts can be beneficial. Advice can be sought from peers and professionals who have faced difficulties, and experiences can be shared to explore alternative solutions.
- Strategic approach: To tackle identified problems, it is important to develop an approach by utilising collected data and available resources. This will help formulate a plan.
- Assessing the urgency and importance of the problem by considering its impact on operations.
- Identify potential solutions: The process of identifying potential solutions involves creating a comprehensive inventory. This inventory, derived from the collected data, includes potential solutions and corrective actions that could address operational issues.
- Practicality evaluation: The analysis of the viability of each prospective solution requires consideration of factors such as financial implications, time constraints, and available resources.
- Optimal course of action: The course of determining the most appropriate solution is based on the solution's practicality and its alignment with goals and priorities.
- Sequential strategy: The task of developing a comprehensive blueprint involves clearly defining the necessary methods.

- An organised framework should consistently track the advancement of the chosen solution, and its efficiency should be evaluated in terms of addressing the identified problem.

2.16 Executing the Result

- Assign roles and responsibilities to each team member to effectively manage the project.
- Provide training and guidance to laboratory personnel to ensure they have the knowledge and skills to contribute effectively to the success of the project.
- Regularly monitor progress by comparing actual results with established timelines and milestones. If there are any deviations from the plan, make adjustments accordingly.
- Maintain lines of communication with team members, management, and other stakeholders involved in the project; this will facilitate addressing any questions, concerns, or issues that may arise during the execution phase.
- Always prioritise safety by adhering to all safety guidelines and preventive measures while carrying out the project.

2.17 Monitoring Progress

- Establish KPIs: Define specific metrics and benchmarks to measure the effectiveness of the action and its impact on outcomes or equipment performance.
- Collect data: Gather data on the relevant KPIs through observation and analysis, both during and after the rendering of solutions.
- Compare results: Compare the collected data to the established benchmarks and targets to assess whether the applied result delivers the desired outcomes and resolves the issue effectively.
- Regular evaluations: The periodic evaluations are not only to assess the competency of embryologists but also to gauge the effectiveness of the troubleshooting process.
- Adjust as required: Based on the empirical data obtained from continuous monitoring, it is recommended to make necessary modifications to the formulated alternative strategies in case the initial solution fails to yield the expected results.

2.18 Communication

- Comprehensive record-keeping on the recognised issue is essential for accelerating the procedure of identifying and executing a suitable action. This will function as a reference point for the purpose of providing information.

- Hold team meetings or training sessions: It is recommended to schedule team meetings or training sessions when the issue at hand is significant or when fixing it leads to changes in SOPs.

- Update SOPs and educational resources: To ensure that everyone is aware of the changes made during the problem-solving course, it is essential to make alterations to SOP training guides. In this way, all relevant information regarding the solutions can be readily available.

- Notify management or regulatory authorities: Whenever deemed necessary, share the outcomes of your troubleshooting exercise with management, regulatory agencies, or any other external stakeholders involved.

- Conduct reviews: These reviews should be scheduled periodically to evaluate the effectiveness of methods and identify areas where improvements can be made.

- Following these steps for communicating results after resolving an issue establishes protocols, promotes internal awareness through meetings/training sessions, updates relevant resources appropriately, and maintains an open dialogue with relevant parties outside the organisation when required.

- It is also essential to involve all team members, and their insights and perspectives can help identify opportunities for improvement and create a sense of ownership and commitment among the team.

- Based on the insights gained from these reviews, input from staff members, and performance metrics, necessary changes should be implemented to enhance the efficiency of the restoration practice.

- It is important to monitor and evaluate these changes' impact on both the process itself and the overall performance of the lab, assessing whether these changes have led to greater effectiveness.

- **Preventive measures:** Preventive measures are crucial to avoid future issues and include the following actions: updating SOPs, regularly providing training for all staff members, and consistently maintaining and performing additional quality control checks.

- Regarding staff training, it is crucial to provide continuous development opportunities, including offering refresher courses to ensure that the staff is updated on the latest advancements in the industry.

- It is important to prioritise the maintenance and monitoring of lab equipment. Scheduling regular maintenance checks is key to identifying any signs of malfunction, which in turn ensures optimal performance and reduces the likelihood of technical issues.

- It is advisable to conduct regular inspections to optimise quality control within the ART technique. Checks should encompass the examination of sample labels, the verification of identities, and the continuous monitoring of lab conditions.

- It is essential to cultivate a culture of communication within the lab. Staff members should be encouraged to voice their concerns regarding any issues that may arise.

- One important task is to monitor and track errors. It is important to keep a record of any errors that occur in the lab in order to analyse this data and identify any recurring problems. This information can be used to take effective preventive measures and make any necessary adjustments to techniques.

- It is important to keep in mind that every troubleshooting scenario is unique and will require specific actions based on the problem at hand.

CHAPTER 2

SUMMARY

- Use materials with known attributes to monitor the effectiveness of the lab and its equipment.
- Conduct consistent internal checks to spot deviations and make necessary corrections.
- Analyse data from control samples to detect irregularities and oversee ongoing patterns.
- Compare outcomes from various labs to discern differences and boost efficiency.
- Distribute samples among different labs to confirm testing methods.
- Promote the sharing of knowledge and expertise within the lab community to ensure a top-tier working environment.
- Engage in shared research endeavours to standardise and enhance techniques across laboratories.
- Examine and rectify any inconsistencies in performance to uphold consistent quality.
- Commit to ongoing progress by frequently updating quality measures considering new data, tech innovations, or industry shifts.
- Case studies: Learn from practical examples of implementing quality control measures in ART laboratory tests.

3

Quality Control Tools: Risk Management

Risk management is a critical element within the operational framework. This active process systematically unveils, examines, and mitigates potential risks that could potentially disrupt the lab's objectives or put patient safety at risk. Risks could stem from various sources, including equipment failure, biohazard exposure, procedural errors, or external factors such as natural disasters. Consequently, risk management aims to ensure that ART labs consistently and reliably deliver high-quality services.

Equipment failure: ART laboratories heavily rely on advanced technological equipment, such as incubators, microscopes, cryopreservation systems, and micromanipulators, all integral to executing successful ART procedures. Despite their sophisticated design, these pieces of equipment are not immune to malfunction or failure. One of the leading causes of equipment failure is inadequate or irregular maintenance, which could result in sudden breakdowns, leading to disruptions in laboratory procedures.

Biohazard exposure: Exposure can occur through direct contact with the specimen, aerosols, spills, or accidental punctures with contaminated sharp objects. Inadequate or inappropriate specimen handling can lead to cross-contamination, potential disease transmission to lab personnel, or even inadvertent specimen mix-ups or loss. It is worth noting that the risk extends beyond just the handling phase, including the storage and disposal of biohazardous materials.

Technical errors: These can range from basic clerical errors in the labelling and identification of samples, which can have devastating consequences like the mishandling of gametes or embryos, to more complex errors in the application of laboratory protocols, including culture media preparation, incorrect timing of the ART procedures, or incorrect assessment of embryos.

External factors: External factors, while less controllable, pose significant risks to ART laboratories. Natural disasters such as earthquakes, floods, or fires can lead to abrupt and significant disruptions in laboratory operations, including equipment damage, loss of power, and potentially irrevocable loss of stored biological specimens. Power outages, even short duration, can compromise the functioning of critical equipment such as incubators and cryotanks. Furthermore, cybersecurity threats, a growing concern in today's digitally dependent world, can lead to the loss of critical data, breach of patient confidentiality, or interference with the electronic operation of lab equipment.

DOI: 10.1201/9781032622736-3

3.1 Risk Assessment

Risk assessment in ART laboratories is an essential process, central to ensuring the safety of both patients and personnel, the integrity of biological specimens, and the efficiency of laboratory procedures.

This process can be systematically carried out using several steps.

Identification of potential risks: It is a meticulous process that requires a complete understanding of laboratory operations, processes, equipment, and workflow. From the handling and storage of gametes and embryos to the functioning and maintenance of laboratory equipment, each component must be analysed for potential hazards.

Following the identification stage, each risk must be thoroughly evaluated through a risk assessment process. The goal here is to estimate the potential impact of each risk and the likelihood of its occurrence. The potential impact of a risk is measured in terms of its possible effects on patient outcomes, lab costs, or disruptions in the lab operation. A tool often used for this evaluation is the risk matrix.

3.2 Risk Matrix

In Table 3.1, each cell in the matrix represents a unique combination of risk likelihood and impact. For instance, 'Frequent delays in routine tasks due to understaffing' is a risk with a likelihood (4) and negligible impact (1), giving it a risk score of 4. Conversely, a 'Mix-up of gametes leading to wrongful embryo transfer' is a risk with almost a certain likelihood (5) and catastrophic impact (5), giving it the highest risk score of 25.

The goal of utilising such a matrix in an ART laboratory is to visually represent risks, aiding in identifying high-priority risks that need immediate attention. This matrix enables lab management to prioritise their mitigation strategies and allocate resources accordingly to address the risks with the highest scores.

The final stage of the risk assessment process involves prioritising the identified risks. In this stage, risks are ranked based on their evaluated potential impact. Prioritisation is critical to effective risk management, as it helps laboratories focus their efforts and resources on mitigating the most severe and probable risks. Risks with high impact are typically addressed first, ensuring that the mitigation strategies offer the highest level of protection and prevention.

3.3 Risk Mitigation

Upon completing a thorough risk assessment, ART laboratories should focus on implementing robust risk mitigation strategies. The ultimate goal of these strategies is to minimise the potential impact of identified risks and enhance the safety, efficacy, and efficiency of lab operations.

TABLE 3.1

Risk Matrix

	Negligible Impact (1)	Minor Impact (2)	Moderate Impact (3)	Major Impact (4)	Catastrophic Impact (5)
Rare likelihood (1)	Short delay in routine sample analysis due to equipment downtime	Mislabelling of noncritical supplies	Breach in the storage protocol of non-critical biological samples	The temporary failure of an incubator, causing potential harm to embryos	The permanent loss of gametes/ embryos due to catastrophic failure of storage system
Unlikely likelihood (2)	A rare allergic reaction to a latex glove by staff	Slight deviation in standard preparation of culture media	Power outage affecting laboratory lighting but not critical equipment	Transient software glitch causing misinterpretation of patient data	Data breach due to a cyber attack exposing sensitive patient information
Possible likelihood (3)	Occasional delays due to high workload	Minor transcription error in noncritical patient documentation	Occasional procedural errors by newly trained staff	Significant deviation from standard culture media preparation	Prolonged equipment failure, causing delays in treatment cycles
Likely likelihood (4)	Frequent delays in routine tasks due to understaffing	Frequent minor procedural errors	Consistent deviation from SOPs by experienced staff	Mislabelling of critical biological samples	Laboratory shut down due to natural disaster
Almost certain likelihood (5)	Continuous delays due to chronic understaffing	Consistent procedural errors due to poor training	Mishandling of biological samples, leading to cross-contamination	Biohazard exposure, causing harm to staff or patients	Mix-up of gametes, leading to wrongful embryo transfer

Remember that this table is a simplified representation. In practice, each level of impact and likelihood and the resulting risk score would be thoroughly defined according to the specific context of each ART laboratory. It is crucial to regularly review and update the risk matrix in line with new technologies, changes in regulation, and new knowledge about potential risks.

Comprehensive equipment management is the first line of defence against the risk of equipment failure. A backup for essential equipment can make the difference between minor disruption and significant losses in the face of unexpected equipment failure.

Regarding biohazard control, SOPs should cover every aspect of specimen handling, from collection to disposal, to prevent cross-contamination, disease transmission, or specimen loss.

Standardisation and documentation of all laboratory procedures are essential to minimise procedural errors. This could involve creating written protocols for every process in the lab, from specimen handling to data recording. These protocols should be routinely reviewed and updated to reflect current best practices. Additionally, staff should receive ongoing training on these standardised procedures to ensure proficiency.

Finally, preparing for external risks requires the development of comprehensive emergency response plans. These plans should envisage a variety of potential disruptions, such as power outages, natural disasters, and cybersecurity attacks, and provide detailed, step-by-step guidance on how to respond to each scenario. A regular drill of these emergency plans can also help ensure a calm, coordinated response when faced with a real-life crisis.

While risk management is crucial in ART laboratories, embedding a risk mitigation culture throughout the organisation is equally important. Promoting this culture can begin with leadership. Laboratory managers and supervisors should demonstrate a commitment to risk management by establishing clear policies, investing in necessary resources for risk prevention and control, and reinforcing the importance of adherence to these policies. This can be achieved through regular communication on risk management topics, incorporation of risk management into strategic planning, and recognition or rewards for exemplary risk management practices.

Training sessions can cover various topics, including identifying and evaluating risks, understanding and applying risk management protocols, and learning from past incidents or near misses. Moreover, a structured boarding process for new staff that emphasises the importance of risk management can lay a strong foundation for their future work.

Furthermore, open communication and a blame-free culture can significantly enhance risk management in ART labs. Staff should feel encouraged to report potential risks or incidents without fear of blame or punishment. This encourages a proactive approach to risk identification and resolution. A nonpunitive approach to errors can also foster a learning culture, allowing the organisation to improve its risk management practices based on past experiences continuously.

Risk mitigation in ART laboratories is a multifaceted process that requires ongoing attention and review. By continuously monitoring and improving these strategies, ART labs can ensure the highest level of patient safety, safeguard precious biological specimens, and maintain operational efficiency under all circumstances.

3.4 Control Charts

Control charts are vital to quality control, as they allow laboratory analysts to monitor performance and to identify any deviations from expected values over time. They help detect variations in a process and determine if they are due to notable causes. In ART labs, control charts are used to ensure quality and maintain standards across processes and parameters.

3.5 Terms in Control Charts

Control chart: A statistical tool that visually represents the changes in a process variable over time. For instance, a control chart can show the lab temperature or the rate of embryonic development. Control charts help assess the consistency and predictability of a process.

Process variables: These refer to characteristics or parameters that are monitored and managed in an ART lab. Examples include temperature, humidity, and embryonic development rate. It is crucial to have control over these variables for reliable outcomes in the lab.

Control limits: These boundaries, determined statistically, define where a process variable is expected to operate under certain conditions. If the variable remains within these limits, it indicates that the process is under control. However, if the value goes beyond these boundaries, it implies the possibility of something happening and may require further investigation.

Common cause variation: This kind of variation refers to the fluctuations that occur in a process due to randomness. These fluctuations do not need any action, as they indicate that the process is operating under statistical control.

Cause variation: Special cause variation indicates uncommon fluctuations in a process. These variations often result from various factors. Variation may suggest that the process is out of control, requiring additional investigation and corrective measures.

Upper control limit (UCL): The upper control limit on a control chart establishes the limit for process variation under normal conditions. If a variable exceeds this limit, it suggests a deviation from the behaviour of the process.

Lower control limit (LCL): In contrast, the lower control limit defines the acceptable limit for process variation. If a variable falls below this limit, it indicates an abnormality.

Centreline: The centreline on a control chart represents either the target value or the process variable. Consistent alignment of the process variable with this line indicates that the process is functioning within its statistical control limits.

3.6 Frequently Used Control Charts

Control charts are tools in QC that analysts use to monitor the performance of laboratory tests over time.

3.7 Types of Control Charts

3.7.1 Levey-Jennings Charts

Levey-Jennings (LJ) charts find application in laboratories for monitoring test accuracy and precision. They were developed by Dr Samuel Levey and Dr Ernest Jennings in the 1950s.

The main purpose of a Levey-Jennings chart is to track QC data for a test or analytical process. It helps identify errors or trends that could indicate issues with the test procedure or instrument used.

A typical Levey-Jennings chart consists of two axes and other elements listed in the following.

- The X axis represents the time or sequence of QC measurements, which can span hours, days, or runs depending on the frequency of testing.
- The Y axis represents the QC values, or measurement results, for an analyte. These values are usually expressed in the same units as the test results.
- The central line represents the desired value for the QC material, typically calculated from a series of control measurements.
- Upper and lower control limits: These limits are established at a distance from the average, usually at +/− 1, 2, or 3 standard deviations (SDs) to define control zones.
- When utilising a Levey-Jennings chart, laboratory staff plot the QC data points on the chart and analyse them for any patterns that might indicate problems with the instrument or process.

3.8 Example of Levey-Jennings Control Chart on ICSI Degeneration

The ICSI degeneration rate refers to the percentage of eggs that deteriorate following the ICSI procedure.

Using a Levey-Jennings chart reveals if a process is statistically under control and identifies systematic variations. In relation to the ICSI degeneration rate, it helps us detect any fluctuations over time. Higher rates of degeneration might suggest issues with the ICSI technique.

To create a Levey-Jennings chart, observations are plotted along with the value (represented by the central line) and control limits (upper and lower). These limits are typically set at distances of +/− 1, 2, and 3 standard deviations from the mean, as shown in Figure 3.1.

The collected data on ICSI degeneration rates is over a period of 10 months.

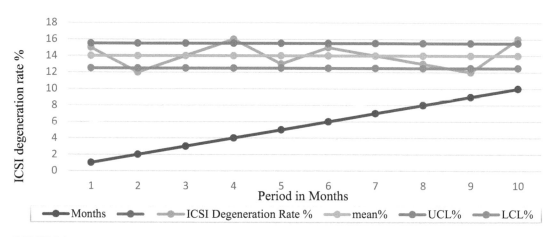

FIGURE 3.1
Example of Levey-Jennings control chart on ICSI degeneration rate.

The average degeneration rate is recorded at 14% with a deviation of 1.5%. Based on this information, the control limits can be calculated as follows:

For +/– 1 deviation

Upper control limit = 15.5%, lower control limit = 12.5%;

For +/– 2 deviations, UCL = 17%, LCL =11%;

And for +/– 3 standard deviations, UCL =18.5%, LCL=9.5%.

Methodology for detecting anomalies: If a data point exhibits a deviation greater than 3 standard deviations from the control limits, it may suggest the presence of a systematic error. Conducting thorough investigations and implementing suitable remedial measures is of the utmost significance. Similarly, if two out of three consecutive data points deviate beyond 2 standard deviations from the control limits, it may indicate a potential trend that could result in the system going out of control. Additionally, if 80% of the data points deviate beyond 1 standard deviation from the control limits, this may suggest the emergence of a discernible pattern in the process.

To ensure reliable results in laboratory tests, Levey-Jennings charts are key tools. These charts plot individual test results against time and help monitor semen analysis, oocyte maturation, and embryo development.

Another useful tool for monitoring shifts over time is cumulative sum (CUSUM) charts. Unlike Shewhart charts, CUSUM charts can detect changes that may not be immediately apparent.

CUSUM charts work as follows:

- Calculate the sum by measuring deviations between the process measurements and a target value (the process mean or desired value).
- Plot the sum on a chart over time to track any shifts or trends.

To analyse the chart, one must search for any patterns or trends that suggest a change in the process. There are characteristics of CUSUM charts to consider, such as the following:

- Sum charts are highly sensitive and can detect even small shifts in the process.
- They are more effective at identifying changes in the process compared to Shewhart charts.
- However, interpreting charts may be more challenging, as they lack precise centrelines and control limits.

Figure 3.2 provides an example of a CUSUM control chart used to monitor pregnancy rates. In this scenario, the target pregnancy rate is set at 40%, which means aiming for 24 pregnancies out of 60 attempts per month. By plotting these deviations over time on a graph with months on the x axis and sum values on the y axis, it can show any significant upward or downward trends. Such trends might indicate a shift in the process and could require further investigation. See Figure 3.2.

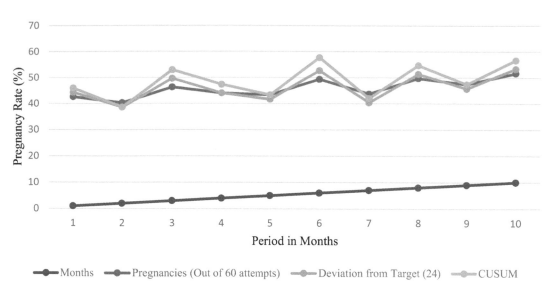

FIGURE 3.2
Example of a CUSUM control chart on pregnancy rate.

3.9 Shewhart Control Charts

Shewhart charts, developed by Walter A. Shewhart, are utilised to monitor the stability of a process and identify factor-related variations. They are also referred to as statistical process control (SPC) charts (Figure 3.3).

Shewhart charts function as described in the following.

- Gather data from the process and calculate the standard deviation.
- Establish control limits based on the process mean and deviation, usually set at +/– 3 deviations from the mean.
- Plot the data points on a chart with the process mean as the line and the control limits as the lower boundaries.

3.9.1 Key Characteristics of Shewhart Charts

- Designed to identify shifts in the process
- Easier to interpret compared to CUSUM charts, with defined centreline and control limits
- Less sensitive than CUSUM charts for detecting shifts in the process

Sum charts are ideal for detecting gradual changes in a process, while Shewhart charts are best suited for spotting sudden shifts. Depending on the specific needs of monitoring and controlling laboratory processes, either or both of these control charts can be selected. Particularly in ART labs, these charts are beneficial for monitoring various stages of the

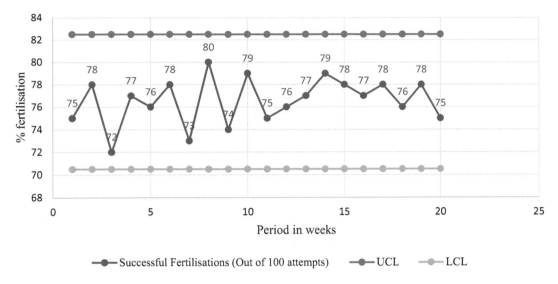

FIGURE 3.3
Example of Shewhart control chart for fertilisation rate.

Note: The UCL and LCL values remain the same across all weeks, as they are calculated from the overall mean and standard deviation of the process.

process. To illustrate, consider the example of monitoring the fertilisation rate. There are 20 samples, each representing the success rate for one week. To establish a control chart for these values, the standard deviation must be calculated. Given that the average fertilisation rate ($\bar{x}$) is 76.5 with a deviation (σ) of 2, the UCL and LCL can be determined. The UCL is calculated as $\bar{x} + 3\sigma$, which in this case would be $76.5 + 32 = 82.5$.

Similarly, the LCL is obtained by subtracting 3σ from $\bar{x}$: $76.5 - 32 = 70.5$.

If any value falls outside these limits, it could suggest that the process is out of control.

Exponentially weighted moving average (EWMA) charts, which are statistical process control tools, are commonly used in labs and industries to monitor and identify shifts in processes. These charts are particularly effective when it is crucial to detect changes in the mean or variability of a process. Unlike SPC tools like Shewhart and CUSUM charts, EWMA charts assign decreasing weights to data points in an exponential manner, making data more sensitive to recent changes.

EWMA is a time series forecasting technique that relies on a moving average, giving importance to the most recent observations. This aspect makes it highly suitable for detecting shifts in a process.

3.10 Explanation of EWMA

- Weighting factor (λ): The weighting factor (lambda) is a value between 0 and 1 that determines how much emphasis is placed on a given data point compared to previous data points. A higher λ value means that recent data points carry weight, causing the EWMA chart to respond faster to process changes.

- Calculation: The EWMA is calculated using the following formula: $EWMA_t = \lambda \times x_t + (1-\lambda) \times EWMA_{t-1}$.
- λ is the weighting factor, a value between 0 and 1.
- x_t represents the data point at time t.

$EWMA_{t-1}$ is the EWMA value from the previous time point $t-1$. To create an EWMA chart, the EWMA values are plotted on the axis against time. Additionally, there is a line representing the process target and upper and lower control limits based on the desired confidence level and process variability. These limits help determine if the process is under control or not.

Interpretation of an EWMA chart involves observing whether the EWMA points remain within the control limits. If the points stay within these limits, it indicates that the process is under control. However, if points go beyond these limits or have random patterns, this suggests that further investigation is needed, as it may indicate an out-of-control process.

One advantage of using EWMA charts is their sensitivity to detecting shifts in the process mean compared to statistical process control tools; this makes them useful for applications where identifying changes is crucial.

> **Data integration**: EWMA charts utilise a moving average that considers both recent observations and past data. This method provides a representation of the process.

Customisation options: The sensitivity of the EWMA chart can be tailored to process requirements or desired responsiveness by adjusting the weighting factor, λ. Limitations of EWMA charts include the following points:

> Large shifts may take longer to be detected with EWMA charts compared to SPC tools like CUSUM charts.
>
> EWMA calculations are more complex than simple moving averages.
>
> EWMA charts are useful for identifying shifts in laboratory processes.

The choice of control chart depends on the type of data being analysed and the specific goals of the laboratory.

3.11 Analysing the Control Chart

Examining trends involves collecting and organising data over a period of time and then representing this data on a graph. This helps to identify recurring patterns or shifts in the data.

Considering point-to-point fluctuations, which represent the variability in any process, significant deviations from data points may indicate a cause of variation that requires further investigation.

- Special cause variation: This kind of variation is not part of the process and can occur due to equipment malfunctions, mistakes made by operators, or changes in the raw materials.

- Run examination: Also referred to as trend analysis, this statistical technique helps identify patterns in data points that consistently go above or below the control limits over a period of time.
- A continuous deviation of data points either above or below control limits for a period suggests a shift or change in the process average, while a gradual alteration indicates a drift. Both scenarios require investigation.
- Cycles and recurring patterns: Keep an eye out for patterns in the data that may indicate a process. Recognising these patterns can help understand how the process behaves and identify sources of variation.
- Control limits: Control limits are determined based on data from the laboratory and are used to monitor parameters such as temperature, pH, and humidity. When a control limit is violated, it signifies that the parameter being monitored is out of control and corrective action needs to be taken.
- Statistical analysis: This involves examining the data to determine if there have been any changes in the process.
- T-test: This test is used to compare the averages of two groups of data to determine if there is a difference. In an ART lab setting, the t-test is applied when comparing the number of oocytes obtained before and after implementing a protocol change.
- ANOVA: ANOVA (analysis of variance) is a method for comparing the averages of data groups. In an ART lab, an ANOVA is used to compare the number of oocytes retrieved from patients or across different days.
- Chi-square test: This method helps identify any relationship between two variables.

3.12 Quality Indicators

Key metrics to assess the performance and effectiveness of ART labs are quality indicators. These indicators provide insights into the laboratory's operations and its quality control system. Important quality indicators include the following:

Turnaround time: This refers to the time that passes between receiving a sample at the laboratory and delivering the test results. It helps gauge how promptly the lab processes samples.

Analytical error rate: This tracks the number of errors that occur during testing. Such mistakes may arise from human oversights, equipment malfunctions, or issues with the materials and supplies used in the lab. A low frequency of errors suggests an effective quality control system, ensuring dependable test outcomes.

Customer satisfaction: In ART labs, customer satisfaction encompasses the positive feelings of clinicians, patients, and other stakeholders involved in the ART process. Satisfaction levels can be assessed through surveys, feedback forms, or direct communication channels. High customer satisfaction signifies that the lab meets users' needs and expectations, while lower satisfaction may indicate areas for improvement.

Embryo development rates: The rate at which embryos progress to the blastocyst stage is an indicator of quality in ART labs. Higher development rates suggest favourable culture conditions and successful fertilisation techniques, while lower rates may raise concerns about laboratory techniques or equipment issues.

By monitoring these quality indicators, ART labs can ensure that their performance aligns with industry standards while continuously striving for improvement.

Success rates: One important factor to consider when evaluating the quality of ART procedures is the rate at which clinical pregnancies are achieved. Monitoring and tracking these success rates allows laboratories to assess their performance and identify areas that require improvement, ultimately increasing the chances of pregnancy.

Evaluation through external quality assessment (EQA): Participating in EQA programmes and proficiency testing provides a measure of a laboratory's performance compared to other labs and industry standards. Consistently performing well in EQA reflects the effectiveness of the laboratory's quality control system.

3.13 Kaizen in ART Labs

Achieving outcomes in ART labs necessitates processes that minimise errors and a commitment to continuous improvement. *Kaizen*, a management philosophy from Japan, embodies the notion of making changes that accumulate over time to bring about significant transformations. It focuses more on progress than sudden and radical transformations.

3.13.1 Principles of Kaizen

Employee empowerment: Kaizen promotes a culture where individuals at all levels are encouraged to contribute ideas for improvement. This fosters a sense of ownership and engagement among lab personnel, creating an environment conducive to innovation and efficiency (Figure 3.4).

Standardisation of procedures: Implementing procedures ensures consistency and minimises errors. By establishing a framework, ART labs enable staff members to perform tasks accurately while enhancing quality control.

Continuous improvement: The core tenet of kaizen is the pursuit of improvement through vigilance and regular evaluation in ART labs. Changes are implemented to optimise processes and outcomes. This commitment ensures that labs stay at the forefront of advancements in technology.

Waste elimination: Kaizen strives to eliminate practices that hinder efficiency. By adhering to these principles, ART labs can achieve improvements in their processes while maintaining standards for reproductive technology advancements. ART labs assess workflows, eliminate steps, and streamline processes to minimise unnecessary time and resource consumption. This optimisation aims to maximise productivity and cost effectiveness.

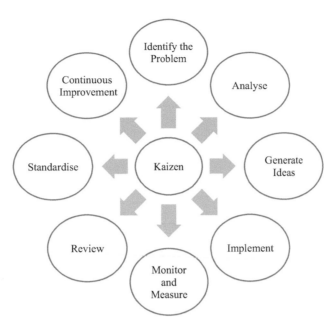

FIGURE 3.4
Diagram of kaizen steps.

Training: Embracing the kaizen philosophy fosters a culture of learning. Regular training sessions empower lab personnel to enhance their skills and stay up to date with emerging technologies and techniques, cultivating a workforce capable of delivering top-notch care.

Incorporating the kaizen philosophy in ART labs drives improvement, resulting in improved processes, reduced errors, and enhanced outcomes.

3.14 Implementation of 6S Methodology in ART Laboratories

ART labs prioritise precision organisation and operational efficiency. One successful approach for enhancing these aspects is the implementation of the Japanese 6S system, which includes a component that focuses on safety.

3.14.1 Understanding the 6S Methodology

The 6S methodology is an approach to organising and standardising workplaces. It consists of six components (Figure 3.5).

Step 1. Sort (*Seiri*): The process begins by separating items. In an ART laboratory setting, this may involve removing equipment or supplies that are not regularly used but take up space.

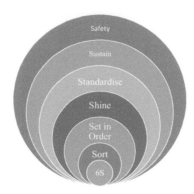

FIGURE 3.5
Diagrammatic representation of 6S principles.

Step 2. Set in Order (*Seiton*): This step requires organising the items in a way that makes them easily accessible and reduces the time spent searching for them. It helps improve efficiency by minimising the time wasted looking for required items.

Step 3. Shine (*Seiso*): Cleaning and maintaining the workspace on a regular basis is crucial. In ART laboratories, this involves taking care of laboratory equipment and keeping the area clean to minimise the risk of contamination.

Step 4. Standardise (*Seiketsu*): Standardising workflows and procedures ensures predictable execution of the three steps. Standard operating procedures play a role in this stage, as they provide instructions for various tasks in the ART lab.

Step 5. Sustain (*Shitsuke*): Sustaining improvements requires discipline and commitment. Regular audits, reviews, and training sessions ensure that the practices of 6S become deeply ingrained in the laboratory's culture.

Step 6. Safety (the sixth 'S'): Safety is an important aspect to consider. Creating a safe work environment in ART laboratories involves managing hazards correctly, handling and storing chemicals, and ensuring proper usage of laboratory equipment.

3.14.2 Benefits of 6S

- **Improved efficiency**: The workflow becomes more efficient through the sorting and organising of items. Laboratory personnel can easily locate the materials they require, minimising wasted time and avoiding disruptions to procedures.

- **Enhanced safety**: A well-maintained and orderly laboratory is inherently safer. By implementing safety measures, the risk of accidents and mishandling of samples can be reduced.

- **Reduced errors**: Standardising processes minimises the likelihood of errors since each step is clearly defined and consistently followed.

- **Increased productivity**: When the workspace is free from clutter, supplies are easily accessible. Moreover, safety protocols are in place, and lab staff can concentrate on their tasks without interruptions or delays.

- **Improved morale**: A clean and organised workspace positively affects the morale and motivation of laboratory personnel. It fosters a sense of pride in their work environment while contributing to job satisfaction.

CHAPTER 3

SUMMARY

- ART labs encounter risks from equipment malfunctions, biohazard exposures, procedural errors, and external threats like natural disasters. They use systematic assessment processes and tools, such as the risk matrix, to manage these risks.

- ART labs manage risks by ensuring equipment upkeep, following stringent SOPs, unifying procedures, and devising detailed emergency response strategies.

- Effective ART lab risk management hinges on a strong risk-focused culture. Leaders should foster this with clear policies, training, transparent communication, and encouraging a proactive, blame-free reporting environment.

- Control charts: Statistical tools that track process variations and detect trends or potential issues.

- Quality indicators: Measurable parameters that assess laboratory performance and help identify areas for improvement.

- Key terms and definitions: Fundamental concepts of control charts and quality indicators.

- Types of control charts: Choice of appropriate control charts for different data types, such as Shewhart charts, CUSUM charts, or EWMA charts.

- Analysis of control chart data: Examination of data points for trends, patterns, or points outside the control limits to determine process stability.

- Statistical tests: Application of chi-square, t-test, and ANOVA to analyse data and assess the effectiveness of quality control measures.

- Regular monitoring: Consistent tracking and evaluation of control charts and quality indicators to maintain high quality standards and to make data-driven decisions for process improvement.

- Kaizen is a Japanese management philosophy for continuous improvement. It empowers employees, standardises procedures, eliminates waste, and promotes a learning culture. ART labs can improve operations, reduce errors, and enhance patient outcomes by integrating kaizen.

- The 6S methodology systematically approaches workplace organisation and standardisation in ART laboratories. It includes sorting, setting in order, shining, standardising, sustaining, and focusing on safety.

- The benefits of implementing 6S include improved efficiency, enhanced safety, reduced errors, and increased productivity.

4

Environmental Monitoring

Environmental monitoring plays a vital role in the dynamic and intricate world of ART laboratories, serving as the cornerstone for achieving successful outcomes for patients. These laboratories operate at the intersection of biology and technology, presenting a unique blend of complexities where even the slightest variations in environmental conditions can significantly impact results.

At the core of an ART lab's environmental monitoring mission lies the task of creating and maintaining ideal conditions for handling delicate biological materials like oocytes and embryos. It is a meticulous process akin to fine-tuning a complex instrument, aiming to orchestrate a harmonious symphony of successful conception and healthy gestation.

The lab diligently evaluates and regulates critical environmental parameters such as temperature, humidity, and air quality. Additionally, vigilance extends to the detection of unseen factors like particulate matter, volatile organic compounds, and microbial contaminants. The objective goes beyond mere detection, involving identifying potential sources of contamination and taking swift, appropriate measures to counteract any risks.

Environmental monitoring goes hand in hand with real-time tracking, enabling quick identification of potential issues and immediate corrective actions to uphold the quality and safety of ART procedures. This unwavering attention aims to optimise the laboratory environment, thereby enhancing the likelihood of successful ART procedures and ultimately contributing to the miracle of life.

Effectively navigating this nuanced terrain requires a deep understanding of the ART laboratory's ecosystem, intricate knowledge of sophisticated equipment, keen observation skills, and an unwavering commitment to patient safety and well-being.

Monitoring equipment: The benefits of environmental monitoring in ART labs are numerous, and monitoring is essential to maintaining a stable and contamination-free environment and safeguarding the viability and development of delicate cells (Figure 4.1).

Key benefits:

- Confirming optimal culture conditions: ART procedures require controlled conditions to foster the best possible outcome.
- Maintaining integrity: Regular monitoring ensures that the lab remains free from external influences that could compromise the quality of the procedures.
- Early detection of potential issues: Environmental monitoring allows for the early detection of problems such as equipment malfunctions, fluctuations in temperature or humidity levels, or the presence of contaminants.
- Ensuring compliance with regulatory standards: ART labs are subject to strict regulatory standards to ensure patient safety and the quality of the procedures.

DOI: 10.1201/9781032622736-4

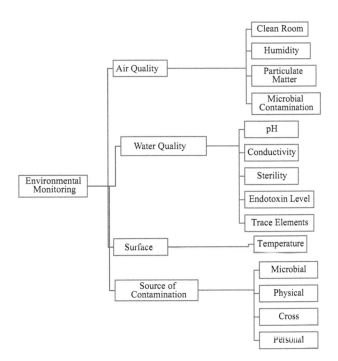

FIGURE 4.1
Factors influencing ART lab environment.

4.1 Sources of Contamination in ART Labs

Airborne particles and the mishandling of materials are sources of contamination. To maintain a safe environment in ART labs, it is vital to implement measures such as controlling air quality, adhering to aseptic techniques, conducting regular cleaning, and monitoring quality control (Figure 4.2).

4.1.1 Microbial Contamination

Microbial contamination in ART labs is a major concern, as it can directly affect the quality and success rate of infertility treatments. The presence of microorganisms in the lab is known as contamination, and these can originate from several sources, such as the air we breathe, water, various surfaces, and laboratory equipment. Interestingly, even lab personnel can inadvertently contribute to this problem, as they can bring these microorganisms into the lab through their clothing, skin, hair, and personal items like mobile phones.

The implications of such contamination are quite severe. Beyond simply compromising the quality of the gametes and embryos, it can also negatively affect the overall success rates of ART procedures, thereby diminishing the chances of conception. Additionally, the risk of infections increases significantly through contamination. It is therefore unsurprising that contaminations often lead to inaccurate lab results, hindering the efficiency of delicate laboratory procedures.

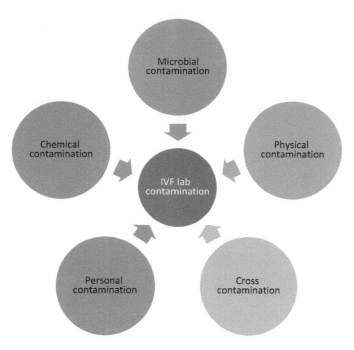

FIGURE 4.2
Primary sources of contamination.

Smartphone contamination: In a revealing study conducted in municipal hospitals of Chongqing, China, researchers investigated the extent of bacterial colonisation on the mobile phones and hands of healthcare workers (HCWs). Of the 111 mobile phones analysed, a staggering 95.5% were found to be contaminated with bacteria.

The most frequently detected strains included *Staphylococcus epidermidis*, followed by *Acinetobacter baumannii* and *Staphylococcus aureus*. The research not only highlighted the risks associated with contamination but also pinpointed the primary factors contributing to this pervasive issue. Notably, frequent phone usage was identified as a significant risk factor, with those using their phones more often exhibiting substantially higher contamination rates—an association underscored by an odds ratio of 8.366. Interestingly, the use of phone covers, which might seem protective, was linked to increased bacterial contamination.

This sheds light on the need for stringent measures to tackle the risk of cross-contamination via contaminated smartphones. Institutions could consider implementing guidelines that mandate healthcare workers clean their smartphones regularly, while individuals should also be encouraged to follow this practice for their safety (Yao et al., 2022).

Prevention of microbial contamination: To prevent contamination, it is important to follow laboratory practices. This includes wearing appropriate attire in the lab, regularly washing hands, and consistently cleaning and disinfecting laboratory equipment and surfaces.

4.1.2 Chemical Contamination

Chemical contamination is another factor that can have an impact on ART procedures. Surprisingly, even disinfectants which are meant to keep the laboratory environment clean can be harmful to eggs and embryos, resulting in reduced viability and lower success rates. Additionally, contamination can arise from plastics and other materials used in the lab, as they may introduce chemicals that adversely affect the outcomes of ART procedures.

Selecting lab disposables is important. This involves consideration of not just the products themselves but also how they are manufactured, and it ensures quality control measures during production. High-quality lab disposables are produced with stringent quality control procedures in place to ensure they meet all required industry standards.

4.1.3 Physical Contamination

There are various sources of contamination in ART labs; one such source is particles and debris that can come from dust, fibres, or other small particles in the air. These particles can settle on surfaces and can be transferred through contact with lab personnel, equipment, or consumables. When this happens, they may contaminate the culture media, compromising the sterility of the laboratory environment. This contamination can also affect the viability of eggs, sperm, and embryos.

Contamination can also occur through laboratory equipment that is improperly cleaned or maintained. Pipettes, incubators, and workstations that are not properly taken care of can introduce contaminants into the lab environment. Additionally, broken glassware or damaged materials can also bring particles into the lab.

Furthermore, consumables used in ART labs can also contribute to contamination if they are non-sterile or expired. Culture media that is not properly maintained or expired pipette tips and Petri dishes pose a risk of introducing contaminants into the lab environment. Regular maintenance and cleaning procedures for both laboratory facilities and equipment are crucial to mitigating this risk.

4.1.4 Personnel Contamination

Personnel themselves can unintentionally contaminate ART labs through their clothing items, skin flakes/hairs/respiratory secretions/fluids, and so on. Personnel contamination refers to the introduction of microorganisms, particles, or other contaminants into the laboratory environment by lab personnel. This compromises the conditions needed for various ART procedures to be successful. Personnel contamination can occur through various means, including the following:

Clothing: Lab coats, uniforms, or even regular street clothes can carry contaminants.

Skin and hair: Skin cells, hair strands, and sebaceous secretions may carry microorganisms or particles that have the potential to contaminate the lab environment.

Respiratory secretions: Coughing, sneezing, or even talking can release droplets containing microorganisms that may settle on surfaces or equipment in the lab.

Other bodily fluids: Touching one's face, nose, or mouth transfers microorganisms to the hands and subsequently contaminates surfaces, equipment, or consumables in the lab.

Personal items: Accessories like jewellery, watches, cell phones, pens, and other personal belongings can harbour contaminants and introduce them into the lab environment.

4.2 Prevention of Personnel Contamination

Personal protective equipment (PPE) should be used as a safeguard for lab workers against threats such as bacteria, viruses, and parasites. The specific PPE required may vary depending on the procedures performed in each laboratory setting. However, common PPE items used in ART labs include gloves, lab coats, hairnets, and face masks.

4.2.1 Hand Hygiene

It is essential for laboratory personnel to thoroughly wash their hands with soap and water for a minimum of 20 seconds. Practising good hand hygiene is the best way to prevent the transmission of infections. Lab staff must diligently clean their hands using soap and water for 20 seconds before and after handling gametes or embryos, using the restroom, or dealing with any potentially contaminated materials. In situations where soap and water are not available, alcohol-based hand sanitisers can be used as an alternative.

4.2.2 Staff Training

It is of the utmost importance that all personnel working in laboratory settings undergo comprehensive training in various techniques; measures to prevent contamination; and proper protocols for handling materials, equipment, and consumables.

Limited access: To mitigate the potential for contamination, it is advisable to restrict the number of individuals authorised to enter the laboratory and to establish appropriate access control measures.

Appropriate laboratory attire: The implementation of regulations pertaining to attire, coupled with the prohibition of certain articles, can effectively contribute to the preservation of a hygienic environment.

Health monitoring: It is strongly advised that laboratory personnel promptly report any instances of illness or symptoms indicative of infection. Policies aimed at prohibiting employees from conducting work within the laboratory setting serve to enhance the overall quality of the working environment.

The maintenance of cleanliness and hygiene is of the utmost importance to ensuring a pristine laboratory environment. It is imperative to diligently clean and disinfect work surfaces, equipment, and communal areas to effectively eradicate any potential contaminants. These practices guarantee a hygienic laboratory setting.

4.3 Cross-Contamination

Cross-contamination in ART laboratories refers to the transfer of microorganisms or other contaminants from one procedure or sample to another. This occurs when materials or equipment used in one ART procedure are not adequately cleaned and disinfected before being used in another procedure.

4.3.1 Prevention of Cross-Personnel Contamination

Cleaning and disinfection: All equipment and materials used in ART procedures must undergo cleaning and disinfection based on established protocols before being used again.

Use of single-use consumables: It is recommended to use pipette tips, culture dishes, and gloves to minimise the risk of cross-contamination.

Segregation of work areas: Allocating workstations for ART procedures is crucial to preventing cross-contamination between them.

Workflow management: Following a defined workflow helps reduce the movement of materials, equipment, and personnel between work areas. This includes designated pathways for sample and material transport as well as assigning specific tasks to individual personnel, thereby decreasing the chances of cross-contamination.

Storage of materials and equipment: Storing materials and equipment in locations separate from workstations helps reduce the risk of contamination. These storage spaces are regularly maintained to ensure cleanliness and sterility.

Training: It is essential to provide training to laboratory staff on laboratory techniques and protocols to effectively prevent cross-contamination.

4.4 Air Quality in ART Labs

Air quality refers to the presence or absence of particles, gases, and microorganisms in the atmosphere. Within ART laboratories, maintaining air quality is vital not only for the well-being of lab personnel but also to create an ideal environment for embryo development while safeguarding against any potential contamination of the embryo culture medium (Figure 4.3).

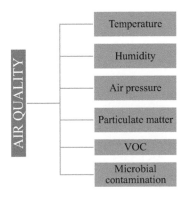

FIGURE 4.3
Air quality contributing factors.

4.4.1 Factors Affecting Air Quality in ART Labs

Personnel and patient activities: The activities carried out by laboratory personnel and patients can contribute significantly to air contamination.

Building location: The location of the building, its geographical surroundings, and various design elements all affect the air quality within ART labs. Elements such as the building envelope, heating, ventilation, and air conditioning (HVAC) systems, and ventilation rates play a role. Buildings situated near roads or industrial areas may experience levels of outdoor pollutants that can potentially penetrate the facility. Additionally, poorly designed HVAC systems may result in poor air circulation, leading to increased concentrations of contaminants in the surrounding environment.

Laboratory equipment and supplies: The type of equipment and supplies used within ART labs can also contribute to air contamination issues. Poorly maintained machinery may inadvertently release particulate matter into the atmosphere.

Ensuring air quality within ART labs requires attention to these various factors to protect both laboratory personnel health as well as successful embryonic development without any risk of contamination.

Cleaning and maintenance: The cleanliness and maintenance practices at ART labs can have an impact on the air quality. If cleaning is inadequate, dust and debris can accumulate, which in turn contribute to the presence of particulate matter in the air. Similarly, if HVAC systems are not properly maintained, dust and other pollutants can build up and circulate in the air, leading to poor air quality.

Chemicals: When disinfectants, solvents, or fixatives are used, there is a possibility of releasing volatile organic compounds (VOCs) into the surrounding environment.

Outdoor air quality: Outdoor pollutants have the potential to enter ART labs through ventilation systems or open windows connected to the air handling unit (AHU), thus contributing to a decline in air quality.

HVAC stands for heating, ventilation, and air conditioning systems. In ART labs, HVAC systems are vital to maintaining optimal air quality and controlling the laboratory environment's temperature, humidity, and air circulation.

Air filters are incorporated into HVAC systems to eliminate particulate matter and other impurities from the air. ART labs frequently employ high-efficiency particulate air (HEPA) filters to effectively remove airborne particles that could potentially harm embryo quality. These filters have a minimum particle removal efficiency of 99.97% for particles larger than 0.3 microns and can filter out an array of airborne contaminants.

Another significant component of HVAC systems in ART labs is air circulation. Air circulation helps maintain a uniform distribution of air and temperature within the laboratory environment to maintain consistent conditions and facilitate the development of embryos. Proper air circulation helps prevent the buildup of contaminants in the air, reducing the risk of contamination of the embryo culture medium.

The optimal air quality in ART labs is contingent upon the appropriate maintenance and monitoring of HVAC systems.

The routine replacement of filters, periodic system inspections, and calibration of temperature and humidity sensors are needed to protect the performance of HVAC systems used in ART laboratories.

Construction: Any construction or renovation activities happening within or near ART labs also play a role in diminishing air quality. These activities generate dust and other particulate matter that is released into the air and spreads throughout the laboratory.

The consequences of poor air quality within ART labs are significant. It can adversely impact embryonic development, reduce fertilisation rates, and increase the risk of fungus contamination. Moreover, it also poses health and safety risks for laboratory personnel and patients.

4.5 Parameters for Air Quality Monitoring

4.5.1 Temperature

In ART labs, the ideal ambient temperature ranges between 22 °C and 25 °C depending on lab requirements and the type of ART procedure being conducted.

To ensure temperature consistency, the strategic placement of temperature sensors allows for real-time monitoring; this enables responses to any fluctuations that may occur. In addition to controlling the temperature, it is crucial to maintain the incubators used for embryo culture at a temperature of 37.0 °C (+/– 0.2), mirroring the human body's natural warmth. Temperature sensors positioned inside the incubators assist in monitoring and maintaining this environment.

The design and maintenance of HVAC systems, insulation of laboratory walls and doors, and the utilisation of incubators and workstations equipped with precise temperature control capabilities ensure the even distribution of temperatures throughout the laboratory setting.

Regularly replacing filters is necessary to prevent dust accumulation or other particulate matter that could disrupt temperature control. Additionally, it is essential for laboratory personnel to undergo training on protocols for regulating temperatures. To ensure temperature regulation in laboratory operations, it is important to establish and follow SOPs.

4.5.2 Humidity Control

Maintaining the levels of moisture in the air, also known as humidity control, is crucial for ART labs. The ideal humidity range should be between 40% and 60%. Fluctuations in humidity can negatively impact embryonic quality due to increased risk of contamination. It is essential to monitor and promptly respond to any changes in humidity levels to effectively control and maintain the desired environment.

4.5.3 Air Pressure Control

The laboratory should be maintained at a higher pressure than the outside environment. This positive pressure helps prevent contaminants from entering the lab. Achieving air pressure control requires well-designed HVAC systems and regular maintenance. Automatic door closures and airlocks also play a role in maintaining this pressure difference.

4.5.4 Particulate Matter

Elevated levels of particulate matter (PM) can have effects on embryonic development and pose risks to lab personnel's health and safety. In ART labs, particle counters are used to detect and count particles based on their size. This measurement focuses on particles ranging from 0.3 to 5 microns. To effectively control particulate matter, it is important to design and maintain HVAC systems that properly utilise air filters and to follow laboratory procedures that minimise the generation of PM.

4.5.5 Monitoring Volatile Organic Compounds

In ART laboratories, monitoring VOCs is given high priority to ensure optimal air quality and to reduce potential risks associated with exposure to harmful chemicals. Acceptable limits for VOC levels in ART labs typically aim to be below 0.5 parts per million (ppm). However, these limits may vary depending on the chemicals being used. The regulations are set by local authorities.

Controlling VOCs involves using products that have VOC content, implementing ventilation systems, and ensuring appropriate storage of chemicals. Specific areas within the lab are designated for chemical storage purposes only and are kept separate from laboratory spaces.

Portable photoionisation detectors (PIDs) are used in ART labs to analyse organic compounds. These handheld instruments measure VOCs by ionising them in the air and measuring the resulting electrical current. While a PID is a specific technique that can detect all types of VOCs, it is not as sensitive or specific as gas chromatography-mass spectrometry (GC-MS).

4.6 Microbial Contaminant Monitoring

The acceptable limits for colony-forming units (CFUs) in ART labs typically aim for less than 500 CFUs per cubic metre of air for bacteria and 50 CFUs per cubic metre for fungi. However, these limits may vary based on the requirements of the ART lab and the type of procedure being performed.

4.7 Strategies for Maintaining Optimal Air Quality

4.7.1 Proper Laboratory Design

To minimise the entry of pollutants, it is beneficial to organise the layout of the laboratory in a way that limits the movement of both materials and personnel. It is recommended to divide the laboratory into sections dedicated to tasks such as oocyte retrieval, embryo culture, and cryopreservation. Including an airlock entrance in the laboratory design helps safeguard against contamination from nearby areas (see Chapter 16).

4.8 Air Filtration Systems

Types of filters: In ART labs, two types of filters are used, prefilters and high-efficiency particulate air filters. Pre-filters, usually made of polyester or fibreglass, effectively capture dust, pollen, and hair. On the other hand, HEPA filters are designed using fibres that create a sort of labyrinth for trapping particles as small as 0.3 microns (Figure 4.4).

Filter efficiency: The efficiency of filters is measured using the minimum efficiency reporting value (MERV) rating scale, which ranges from 1 to 20. A higher MERV rating indicates an effective filter. For HEPA filters in ART labs, it is recommended to choose a filter with a rating of 14 or higher. Filters with this rating can capture over 99.995% of particles as small as 0.3 microns, ensuring effective removal of airborne contaminants from the laboratory.

Air exchange rate: The air exchange rate is the number of times the air inside the laboratory is replaced with clean, filtered air per hour. A higher air exchange rate means that the air inside the lab is refreshed more frequently. ART labs' recommended air exchange rate is 15–20 air changes per hour to ensure that the air inside the lab is filtered and replaced frequently enough to maintain a clean environment.

Filtration system design: The air handling system should be balanced so that air flows from clean to dirty areas. The system's design also considers the laboratory's layout, procedures, and the number of people working in the lab.

4.9 Positive Air Pressure

Entry points: Ensuring consistent air pressure is essential to prevent outside air from infiltrating. In the laboratory, particular focus should be on potential entry points such as doors, windows, and vents.

Airlocks: Airlocks play a role in maintaining pressure and preventing contaminated air from escaping.

4.10 Regular Cleaning and Maintenance

To maintain a well-functioning laboratory, it is recommended to establish a cleaning schedule that includes tasks such as wiping down work surfaces and equipment with solutions. Monthly tasks should focus on maintaining and cleaning air ducts, filters, and exhaust fans.

FIGURE 4.4
Photograph showing clean and contaminated laminar air flow prefilter.

4.11 Cleaning Agents

When selecting cleaning agents for an ART lab, it is crucial to use formulations specifically designed for laboratory environments. These agents should not leave any residue or emit VOCs. Always follow the manufacturer's instructions when using cleaning agents, ensuring they are used at the recommended concentration for effectiveness.

> **Maintenance of Equipment:** It is important to perform maintenance tasks such as cleaning, replacing filters, calibrating equipment, and conducting inspections. Keeping a logbook to document these activities helps ensure that they are completed successfully and regularly.

4.12 Sterilisation Methods

Heat Sterilisation: In this heat sterilisation process, high temperatures are used to sterilise equipment, work surfaces, and laboratory areas. Autoclaving is the most commonly used heat sterilisation method, where steam under pressure reaches temperatures up to 121 °C.

Chemical Sterilisation: Chemicals like ethanol and glutaraldehyde are used in sterilisation to eliminate microorganisms. Unlike heat sterilisation, which requires high temperatures, chemical sterilisation is performed at temperatures suitable for materials sensitive to heat. However, this method may require exposure periods for sterilisation and could leave residues on the materials that need additional rinsing.

Radiation Sterilisation: Gamma rays, UV light, or electron beams are employed in radiation sterilisation to kill microorganisms. This method is useful for materials that cannot tolerate temperatures or chemical treatments. Nevertheless, radiation sterilisation demands equipment and may incur higher costs compared to other methods.

4.13 Use of Low-VOC Materials and Chemicals

To ensure the safety of embryo development, it's imperative for ART laboratories to use materials and chemicals that minimise the emissions of volatile organic compounds. This means choosing paints, adhesives, and flooring materials with low or no VOC emissions. Additionally, selecting cleaning agents and chemicals that have reduced VOC emissions is crucial to maintaining air quality and preventing respiratory irritants. However, it is important to note that while using low-VOC materials and chemicals is necessary, proper ventilation and air exchange should not be overlooked. Adequate air exchange is essential for bringing in clean, filtered air and swiftly removing any contaminants. To uphold quality and safety standards in the laboratory, personnel must receive training on cleaning procedures, sterilisation processes, and equipment maintenance through SOPs. These protocols also address contamination control guidelines for handling materials and biological waste.

Reporting: It is the responsibility of laboratory personnel to promptly report any incidents or deviations from protocols to their lab manager. Immediate reporting minimises the risk of negative consequences and allows for the implementation of appropriate measures.

4.14 Real-Time Monitoring Devices

Parameters: Real-time air quality monitoring devices measure factors such as temperature, humidity, air pressure, particulate levels, carbon dioxide, and VOCs.

Sampling methods: Real-time air quality monitoring devices employ sampling techniques including active or continuous methods.

Sensor technology: The accuracy and precision of measurements in real-time air quality monitoring devices are influenced by the sensor technology employed.

Real-time data and alerts: The data collected by the sensors is transmitted instantly to a monitoring system, where it is analysed and compared against limits. When a parameter exceeds its designated boundaries, it activates an alert. Relevant personnel are notified via email, text message, or an alarm system.

Calibration: To calibrate air quality monitoring devices, it is common practice to use certified calibration gases that contain known concentrations of pollutants. The sensors in the monitoring device are exposed to the calibration gas, and their readings are compared to the known gas concentration.

User interface: One effective approach is to present the data in a simple manner that is easy to understand. It is vital to give users access to both the data itself and the ability to track trends over time. Furthermore, it is important for the interface to provide users with the ability to customise their thresholds and notification preferences.

4.15 Data Logging and Reporting

While local servers grant enhanced control over data storage, cloud-based systems offer advantages in terms of scalability and accessibility. Irrespective of the storage method selected, it remains imperative to encrypt data, ensuring protection against unauthorised access. Reporting plays a role in ensuring compliance with requirements and maintaining transparency with stakeholders. Data needs to be reported to highlight parameters being monitored, conditions encountered, and any corrective actions taken. Reports can be generated either automatically or manually using software that leverages predefined templates and thresholds for automated reporting purposes.

For monitoring and control of parameters, it is essential to integrate continuous monitoring systems with building management systems and HVAC systems. This integration is made possible through the use of protocols like Modbus or BACnet, which facilitate communication between devices manufactured by companies.

4.16 Scheduled Assessments of Different Air Quality Parameters

Microbial air sampling is a technique used to identify and measure microorganisms in the air.

The settle plate method aids in detecting particles and microorganisms that settle onto agar plates. It is a cost-effective approach that provides insights into the types and quantities of microorganisms found in the air. However, it has its limitations. For an accurate assessment of air quality, it's important to take samples while accounting for factors like air currents, temperature, and humidity, as well as ensuring proper placement of settle plates. Adhering to the manufacturer's guidelines for placing the settle plates is key to achieving reliable results. Active air sampling is a technique that involves using an air sampler to draw in air either through a filter or an agar plate. The collected sample is then incubated to identify and count the number of colony-forming units effectively detecting microorganisms suspended in the air.

Impaction sampling is a method for detecting both larger and smaller particles as well as microorganisms. Various impaction samplers exist, each with its distinct advantages and disadvantages. In laboratories, the samplers used are Andersen, and reuter centrifugal sampler (RCS). The Andersen sampler is a single-stage impactor designed to collect particles ranging from 0.3 to 10 micrometres in size. The RCS sampler is a stage impactor capable of collecting particles between 0.1 and 10 micrometres in size. The Reuter centrifugal sampler serves as a high-volume impactor that can collect particles sized from 0.1 to 100 micrometres.

Choosing sampling locations: Sampling locations are chosen based on a risk assessment of the laboratory environment, ensuring that the samples accurately represent the lab's air quality. High-risk areas where procedures are performed and aerosol generation occurs are more likely to be included, as well as low-risk areas with no procedures.

Sampling frequency: The frequency at which air samples are taken depends on factors such as the types of ART procedures being conducted, the sensitivity of the laboratory, and any regulatory requirements in place. For example, laboratories involved in IVF may need to conduct air sampling every month.

Trend analysis: Analysing patterns and carefully evaluating data over time can determine if the current sampling frequency is adequate and can help to assess whether any adjustments are needed to ensure monitoring. To ensure control of counts and particle levels, it is crucial to establish specific thresholds or boundaries. These limits should be determined based on guidelines or industry standards.

Particle counters: Particle counters are commonly employed to measure the levels and dispersion of particles in the atmosphere.

Calibration: To ensure accurate measurements, it is advisable to calibrate particle counters. Calibration can be accomplished through the use of calibration particles or other techniques for calibration purposes.

Sampling locations: Sampling locations are selected based on the likelihood of contamination. High-risk areas refer to those where procedures are performed, while low-risk areas are those where no procedures take place.

Sampling frequency: The frequency at which we sample depends on the risks involved and compliance with requirements. Certain regulations mandate particle counting, while others require monitoring.

4.17 VOC Measurement Devices

Particle size range: In cleanrooms, particle counters should have the capability to measure particles ranging from 0.5 to 5 microns. This size range is particularly important to maintaining the desired cleanliness levels in cleanroom environments.

Portable VOC measurement devices known as photoionisation detectors are utilised to detect and measure the concentration of compounds in the air. PIDs are designed to be lightweight, portable, and user friendly, making them highly suitable for on-site monitoring and swift air quality screening in ART labs.

The functioning of PIDs involves generating high-energy ultraviolet light through a lamp, which then causes the ionisation of VOCs present in the air. This process leads to the creation of charged ions and free electrons. The charged ions are subsequently collected on a charged electrode, generating an electric current that is directly proportional to the concentration of VOCs in the air. This current is displayed on a screen, enabling real-time monitoring of VOC concentrations.

4.18 Third-Party Evaluations and Certification

Third-party evaluations and certifications offer an impartial evaluation of the air quality within ART laboratories.

The International Organisation for Standardisation (ISO) has established air quality standards for ART labs. These standards, such as ISO 14644 and ISO 18562, focus on ensuring cleanroom environments and assessing emissions from devices. When it comes to certification, the ISO certification process involves evaluating how a laboratory adheres to ISO standards. This evaluation includes reviewing documents, conducting on-site inspections, and testing air quality parameters.

The certification process typically consists of steps that a laboratory needs to follow.

1. Initial assessment: The laboratory undergoes an evaluation to identify any areas where it may not meet ISO standards. Based on this assessment, a plan is developed to achieve certification.

2. On-site evaluation: An independent auditor visits the laboratory to assess its environment and determine compliance with ISO standards. During this visit, the auditor carefully reviews documentation related to air quality monitoring and corrective actions.

3. Corrective actions: If any noncompliance issues are identified during the evaluation, the laboratory must create and implement a plan to effectively address these issues.

4. After implementing the action plan, a follow-up evaluation is conducted to ensure that all non-compliance issues have been effectively resolved.

5. Certification is granted to a laboratory that successfully meets all ISO requirements and standards. This certification serves as recognition of the lab's dedication to delivering results while continuously improving its operations in accordance with established standards.

Complying with ISO standards entails meeting criteria related to monitoring air quality, maintaining documentation, and taking actions when necessary.

Maintaining records regarding air quality monitoring, corrective actions taken, and other relevant requirements is crucial for laboratories. To address any compliance issues identified during the certification process, it is essential to develop and implement measures for resolution.

Regular audits should be conducted to ensure compliance with ISO standards. Additionally, personnel should receive training updates and make adjustments to the laboratory environment and procedures as needed.

4.19 Cleanroom Classifications and Standards

The ISO cleanroom standards encompass a collection of internationally recognised standards that establish specific criteria for cleanrooms, clean air devices, and the testing and monitoring of cleanroom environments.

The two primary standards for cleanrooms are ISO 14644 and ISO 14698.

ISO 14644: ISO 14644 defines cleanroom classifications based on the maximum allowable concentration of airborne particles. The standard uses a logarithmic scale to quantify particle density, with each class defining a specific upper limit on the number of particles present per cubic metre of air.

The ISO cleanroom classification system ranges from Class 1 to Class 9, with Class 1 being the most stringent and Class 9 being the least stringent (Table 4.1).
ISO 14698 is a set of guidelines that focus on controlling biocontamination in cleanrooms.

Cleanroom classifications: Cleanrooms are categorised based on the concentration of airborne particles within them. The ISO cleanroom standards and the US Federal Standard 209E are two systems utilised for classifying cleanrooms.

4.20 US Federal Standard 209E

US Federal Standard 209E was formulated by the US federal government in 1963 as a comprehensive directive for cleanrooms. Cleanroom standards are established to provide guidance for the design, operation, and maintenance of cleanrooms. These standards are designed to ensure that the air quality, airflow, filtration, and overall functionality of cleanrooms meet the specified requirements.
The following are examples of cleanroom standards around the world.

ISO 14644: This internationally recognised standard establishes norms for cleanroom design, operation, and maintenance according to ISO cleanroom classifications. It covers aspects such as air cleanliness, pressure differentials, temperature, and humidity control to ensure that environments meet predetermined levels of cleanliness and sterility.

USP <797>: This standard, set by the United States Pharmacopoeia, focuses on compounding guidelines. It includes requirements for cleanroom design, air quality management, personnel training, and monitoring. The goal is to prevent harm to patients by avoiding contamination (particulate) variations in compounded preparations' intended strength or using ingredients of inappropriate quality.

BS 5295: This is a British standard that defines cleanroom classification based on the number of particles per cubic meter at specific particle sizes.

EU GMP guidelines: These guidelines, which are mandated by the European Union, set out the standards for ensuring the cleanliness of manufacturing products. These guidelines include requirements for maintaining cleanroom environments in production.

TABLE 4.1

The Maximum Allowable Particle Concentration for Each Class

Class	Maximum Allowable Particle Concentration
Class 1	10 particles/m³ of size 0.1 µm or greater
Class 2	100 particles/m³ of size 0.1 µm or greater
Class 3	1,000 particles/m³ of size 0.1 µm or greater
Class 4	10,000 particles/m³ of size 0.1 µm or greater
Class 5	100,000 particles/m³ of size 0.1 µm or greater
Class 6	1,000,000 particles/m³ of size 0.1 µm or greater
Class 7	352,000 particles/m³ of size 0.5 µm or greater
Class 8	3,520,000 particles/m³ of size 0.5 µm or greater
Class 9	35,200,000 particles/m³ of size 0.5 µm or greater

4.21 External Laboratory Assessments

External evaluations conducted by organisations such as the International Laboratory Accreditation Cooperation (ILAC), the American Association for Laboratory Accreditation (A2LA), and the College of American Pathologists (CAP) play a role in assessing laboratories. While these assessments are typically voluntary, certain regulatory agencies may require them as part of licencing or accreditation procedures.

During a laboratory assessment, experts in laboratory quality management and technical competence conduct on-site inspections to review aspects of the laboratory operations. This includes examining laboratory procedures, equipment, and personnel qualifications and conducting sample testing to evaluate performance. Based on their findings, the assessors assign a score or rating that reflects how well the laboratory meets standards.

Completing an assessment can lead to accreditation or certification for laboratories, which serves as recognition of their competence and commitment to quality.

4.21.1 Benefits of External Laboratory Assessments

A significant advantage of laboratory assessments is their ability to evaluate the performance of a laboratory in meeting established quality standards. The evaluation is conducted by external assessors who possess specialised knowledge in laboratory quality management.

Furthermore, these assessments serve the purpose of identifying areas in which enhancements can be implemented within the laboratory's processes, procedures, and equipment. The provision of this valuable feedback enables laboratories to consistently improve their operations and ensures compliance with rigorous quality standards.

4.22 External Assessments in India

In India, there is an organisation called the Indian Society for Assisted Reproduction (ISAR) that grants accreditation to ART labs. ISAR is a group dedicated to promoting research and education in the field of reproduction in India. To receive ISAR accreditation, IVF labs undergo an evaluation of their facilities, equipment, procedures, and staff qualifications. The accreditation process includes on-site inspections and assessments of the lab's quality control measures and documentation. The lab's performance is evaluated based on outcomes, laboratory procedures, quality control practices, and safety measures.

Aside from ISAR accreditation, ART labs in India also have the option to seek accreditation from recognised organisations such as the Joint Commission International (JCI) or the ISO. These organisations set standards for quality healthcare and may be relevant for IVF labs involved in international research or that serve international clients.

Furthermore, there is another accrediting body called the National Accreditation Board for Hospitals and Healthcare Providers (NABH), which provides accreditation for ART clinics in India. The NABH accreditation programme follows guidelines that cover aspects of ART clinics. Similar to ISAR accreditation, this process involves physical inspections and reviews of quality control procedures and documentation at the clinic. NABH accreditation holds significance, as it represents excellence in assisted reproduction within India.

NABL, which stands for the National Accreditation Board for Testing and Calibration Laboratories, oversees the accreditation process for testing and calibration laboratories in India. This organisation plays a role in maintaining India's quality infrastructure by upholding technical expertise within these facilities.

4.23 Air Quality Control and Improvement

A practical approach to air quality management typically involves the execution of monitoring and testing protocols, preventive strategies, and remedial actions.

4.23.1 Monitoring and Testing

Specialised equipment is employed for testing the laboratory environment by measuring air quality levels. The frequency and extent of these tests are customised to suit the specific needs and treatments of each laboratory.

4.23.2 Preventive Measures

In addition to monitoring, a comprehensive plan for air quality management should include strategies to prevent potential contamination; this could involve implementing cleaning protocols for surfaces, equipment, and tools or utilising high-efficiency air filters that can effectively trap particles.

4.23.3 Corrective Actions

Despite taking preventive measures, there may still be instances where air quality issues arise. When this happens, it is essential to have an action plan ready; this might include improving ventilation systems using air purifiers or additional filters or temporarily suspending treatments until the air quality problem has been fully resolved.

4.24 Identifying and Addressing Sources of Contamination

Common sources of contamination can be chemicals, microorganisms, and particulate matter that originate from equipment, cleaning agents, or even lab personnel. To minimise these risks, it is vital to regulate usage in the lab environment, choose cleaning agents carefully, and provide thorough training to staff regarding proper cleaning procedures.

4.25 Advanced Air Purification Technologies

4.25.1 Ultra-Low Particulate Air Filters

Incorporating air purification technologies adds to existing strategies for managing air quality and helps to safeguard conditions within ART laboratories. One such technology is ultra-low particulate air (ULPA) filters, which are even more effective than HEPA filters in removing particles from the air. ULPA filters have the ability to eliminate up to 99.999% of particles measuring 0.12 microns or larger. They are commonly utilised in environments that demand a high level of air quality, such as cleanrooms.

4.25.2 Activated Carbon Filters

Another essential tool for purifying the air are activated carbon filters. These filters excel at removing VOCs and other gaseous pollutants from the surrounding atmosphere. By adsorbing pollutants onto activated carbon with its structure and high surface area, these filters effectively enhance air quality.

4.25.3 Photochemical Oxidation

Photochemical oxidation stands out as a technology that employs light and titanium dioxide to break down organic pollutants present in the air. This technique significantly reduces levels of VOCs, contributing to cleaner and healthier indoor environments.

4.26 Maintaining Air Quality

4.26.1 Minimising Movement and Foot Traffic

To reduce the risk of contamination, it is important to minimise foot traffic and personnel movement within the lab. We recommend providing training to laboratory personnel on the significance of being mindful of their movements. Sudden movements can create turbulence, worsening the spread of contaminants. Establishing zones for both personnel and equipment movement is also recommended.

4.26.2 Adhering to Protocols and Guidelines

Regularly reviewing and updating protocols based on scientific advancements and regulatory mandates is highly recommended.

4.26.3 Regular Cleaning and Disinfection

Maintaining air quality involves cleaning and disinfecting laboratory surfaces and equipment.

4.26.4 Proper Waste Management

It is vital to ensure the disposal of waste by using designated containers for different types of waste. Educating staff on waste disposal procedures is essential, including the use of sharps containers, biohazard bags, or other appropriate waste containers that comply with requirements.

4.27 Water Quality Management

pH: In ART labs and incubators, the pH of the water is closely monitored. Maintained within a specific range, this ensures that the environment for embryonic development is optimal. The recommended pH range for incubator water is typically between 7.2 and 7.4; any deviations from this range can have effects on the pH of the culture medium, which in turn can lead to lower fertilisation rates and lower embryo quality.

Conductivity: Conductivity measures the ability of water to conduct electricity and serves as an indicator of water purity to prevent interference with embryonic development. For incubator water, it is generally recommended to maintain conductivity levels below 3 microsiemens per centimetre (µS/cm). High conductivity can result in an accumulation of ions in the culture medium, which negatively affects embryonic development and viability.

Sterility: Maintaining sterility helps prevent contamination and also aids in avoiding any potential chemical reactions or changes in pH that may be triggered by bacteria or other microorganisms.

Endotoxin levels: Endotoxins are lipopolysaccharides found in the membrane of gram-positive bacteria, and they can trigger inflammatory responses in embryos. Water used in incubators for purposes typically contains less than 0.25 endotoxin units (EU)/ml.

Trace elements: For embryo development, trace elements like copper, zinc, and manganese are necessary. Available water already contains levels of these trace elements to ensure optimal embryo development.

Storage: When storing water for incubators, it is important to use containers and keep them at the right temperature while also keeping them away from potential sources of contamination.

Shelf life: Using expired water negatively affects the water quality and has an impact on gametes and embryos.

4.28 Surface Monitoring and Control

Monitoring and controlling surface conditions are essential components of laboratory operations and management. The establishment of a controlled environment is of utmost importance to uphold the quality and viability of gametes and embryos.

4.29 Cleanroom Design

ART laboratories have been purposefully designed as cleanrooms to mitigate the potential hazards associated with contamination.

Positive pressure: The differential pressure mechanism ensures that any potential leaks or gaps will result in air flowing outward, effectively preventing the entry of contaminants. Cleanrooms utilise air handling units and air volume systems to regulate airflow and maintain pressure.

Airflow management: Laminar flow hoods ensure a flow of HEPA-filtered air over the workspace, creating a controlled airflow pattern that minimises turbulence and reducing the risk of cross-contamination between workstations. Additionally, air showers are utilised at entrance and exit points to remove particles from personnel and materials before they enter the cleanroom.

Proper room layout: A properly designed room layout aims to minimise the movement of personnel and materials, thereby reducing the risk of contamination. Designing the layout involves placing workstations, equipment, and storage areas to optimise efficiency.

Surface materials: Countertops and work surfaces in cleanrooms often use steel due to its resistance to corrosion and ability to withstand cleaning agents. Non-chemical-resistant and easy-to-clean surface materials are also considered for maintaining cleanliness. Tempered glass is a good choice for walls and windows, as it provides durability.

Temperature control and light: Cleanrooms require adequate lighting to facilitate work. Typically, LED lights are preferred as they generate minimal heat and are energy efficient.

Access control: In the context of access control, it is crucial to implement measures that limit and manage the ingress and egress points within controlled environments. This objective can be accomplished by utilising access systems such as keycards or biometric authentication methods.

4.30 Cleaning and Disinfection Protocols

Maintaining a laboratory environment requires attention to cleaning and disinfection protocols. While specific guidelines may vary, it is important to follow certain advice.

To effectively disinfect surfaces, it is recommended to use either 70% ethanol or a quaternary ammonium compound. These substances target the microorganisms found in laboratory settings.

After the disinfection process, it is essential to dry surfaces using paper towels. Proper disposal of these towels is crucial to preventing cross-contamination. It is best to avoid using towels or cloths, as they can harbour microorganisms and contribute to contamination.

To create a laboratory setting, it is advisable to schedule deep-cleaning sessions. Additionally, it is important for face masks to adequately cover both the nose and mouth areas. Masks must be replaced when they become saturated. As a precaution against hair shedding onto surfaces, wearing hairnets is strongly recommended since this can help prevent contamination.

4.31 Surface Monitoring Techniques

One way to identify contamination is through an inspection, which is a simple and cost-effective technique. However, it is important to note that this method may not always detect chemical residues in tiny amounts that are invisible to the naked eye or present in low concentrations.

For a quantitative approach to detecting organic residues on surfaces, ATP bioluminescence can be used. This method is effective in identifying chemical residues as well and is more sensitive than visual inspection. However, ATP bioluminescence tends to be more expensive due to the need for equipment.

Another option is testing, which involves collecting samples from surfaces using swabs or contact plates and analysing them in a laboratory. In this way, we can determine if there are microorganisms present on the surfaces being tested. The results of these tests help us evaluate the cleanliness of the surfaces and assess the risk of contamination or infection.

4.32 Workstation Organisation and Workflow

To maintain a clean environment and reduce the risk of cross-contamination, it is recommended to implement workflow patterns involving the movement of materials and equipment from clean areas to dirty areas.

To minimise the chances of contamination, it is advisable to assign personnel and equipment to specific areas. Avoiding movement between areas can help mitigate the possibility of cross-contamination. It is important to sanitise both personnel and equipment after their use when transitioning between different zones. Transparent surface monitoring and control protocols should be established, with all staff members encouraged to follow them. Periodic audits should also be conducted to assess the effectiveness of surface monitoring and control practices.

CHAPTER 4

SUMMARY

- Environmental monitoring is critical for quality control in ART labs, consisting of the sources of contamination, air quality management, water quality management, and surface monitoring techniques.

- Sources of contamination in ART labs include microbial, chemical, physical, personnel, or cross-contamination.

- Maintaining optimal air quality is crucial to the success of ART procedures and strategies for achieving proper laboratory design, air filtration systems, positive air pressure, regular cleaning, maintenance, use of low-VOC materials, chemicals, personnel training, and protocol adherence.

- Water quality management is essential for maintaining a sterile environment in ART labs, with regular testing and strict water storage, handling, and use protocols.

- Surface monitoring techniques using swabs, contact plates, and ATP testing are needed to maintain optimal surface quality in ART labs, with personnel adhering to strict cleaning protocols.

- Best practices for maintaining environmental quality in ART labs include regular monitoring, testing, implementing preventative measures, identifying and addressing sources of contamination, and routine maintenance of environmental monitoring systems.

- Advanced air purification technologies, such as UV germicidal irradiation, enhance air quality control in ART labs.

- External evaluations for ISO cleanroom classifications and standards reassure patients and stakeholders regarding the quality of environmental controls in ART labs.

- Ultimately, strict environmental monitoring protocols are fundamental for the safety and success of ART procedures, contributing to overall patient satisfaction.

5

Equipment Maintenance:
Types of Equipment Used in ART Labs

ART labs employ a variety of equipment to aid in the handling, manipulation, and storage of gametes and embryos. It is critical to ensure that these instruments are properly maintained and calibrated for the operation of an ART lab.

5.1 Equipment for Andrology

Centrifuges play a role in andrology laboratories, as they assist in the separation of sperm from plasma and other cellular debris. There are two techniques used for this process: density gradient centrifugation and the swim-up method. Each technique offers distinct advantages depending on the desired outcome.

Rotor inspection and maintenance: Regular inspection of centrifuge rotors detects any signs of cracks, corrosion, or imbalance. This step is crucial, as damaged rotors can result in failures during operations. The manufacturer's guidelines should be followed to clean and lubricate rotors and moving parts to extend their lifespan and ensure functionality.

Temperature control system: Temperature plays a role in sperm processing, as it directly impacts sperm viability and motility. Periodically testing the temperature control system of the centrifuge according to the manufacturer's recommendations can confirm correct functioning. If any inconsistencies or issues arise, they must be addressed promptly to maintain operating conditions.

Speed calibration and general maintenance: Accurate speed settings are essential for obtaining consistent results when separating sperm.

It is important to adjust the speed settings of the centrifuge using a tachometer or other recommended tools for calibration purposes.

5.2 Computer-Assisted Sperm Analysis Systems

Computer-assisted sperm analysis (CASA) systems rely on computer algorithms to provide unbiased results when evaluating sperm motility and morphology. These systems generate data on sperm parameters, allowing for accurate comparisons between samples and tracking changes over time. CASA systems also have the advantage of analysing samples, enabling high throughput capabilities.

DOI: 10.1201/9781032622736-5

In research settings and clinical trials, it is crucial to establish standardisation protocols across laboratories to ensure that results are comparable across institutions. Additionally, CASA systems often incorporate software that simplifies data storage and retrieval, streamlines record-keeping procedures, and enhances data management effectiveness. This contributes to maintaining quality control standards.

To ensure performance, it is essential to calibrate the system using samples with known properties that confirm measurement precision. Regular cleaning and maintenance of the microscope, stage, and camera according to the manufacturer's recommendations are also necessary.

Periodic validation of CASA system performance involves comparing its findings with periodic evaluations as a benchmark.

5.2.1 Software Updates

To optimise the performance of the CASA system, it's advisable to upgrade its software with the newest algorithms, enhancing its capabilities.

> **Emerging tools for semen analysis:** AI-based semen analysis tools employ sophisticated image processing and artificial intelligence to assess semen samples with increased accuracy. These tools capture high-definition images of the samples, and AI algorithms subsequently analyse them for sperm count, morphology, and motility. Additionally, the system can evaluate advanced parameters, such as path velocity and DNA fragmentation levels. The findings are aggregated into comprehensive reports for fertility experts. The primary benefits of these instruments encompass improved accuracy, efficiency, and the capability to offer an in-depth analysis, diminishing the human error and subjectivity present in traditional methods. Nevertheless, appropriate validation and calibration are vital for ensuring peak performance.

5.3 Embryology Equipment

5.3.1 Laminar Flow Hoods

Laminar flow hoods are used in a controlled and sterile environment for purposes such as preparing culture media and working with gametes and embryos. Their main objective is to protect these samples from contamination by utilising HEPA filters.

5.3.2 Vertical Laminar Flow Hoods

Vertical laminar flow hoods operate by directing a stream of air onto a work area; this creates a controlled environment that minimises impurities, making it suitable for handling samples. The hood's intake system consists of a prefilter that efficiently removes particles, followed by a HEPA filter that eliminates bacteria and viruses. The purified air is then channelled downward into the area, creating a germ-free environment. The rate at which the air flows in this system is carefully controlled to prevent any disturbance that could lead to contamination while still effectively removing any particles from the work surface.

Horizontal laminar flow hoods are designed specifically to protect samples from contamination. They achieve this by directing the airflow across the designated work surface. This design effectively prevents contaminants from entering, ensuring the integrity of the samples.

To maintain effectiveness in eliminating contaminants, it is necessary to replace prefilters and HEPA filters. The frequency of replacement may vary depending on filter type and usage.

Regularly measuring the airflow rate within the hood is crucial to ensuring it falls within given limits. An anemometer can be used as a method for achieving this goal.

Performance qualifications (PQs) are recommended to verify that the system functions properly. PQ testing assesses whether the hood maintains desired airflow rates, particle counts, and sterility levels.

5.3.3 Incubators

Incubators are essential in ART labs, as they play a role in IVF procedures and other ART techniques.

The following are the main types of incubators commonly used in IVF labs:

CO_2 incubators: These are the incubators used in IVF labs. They create an environment by regulating the temperature, usually set at 37 °C (body temperature), and maintaining a carbon dioxide (CO_2) concentration, typically around 5%–6%. This CO_2 concentration is crucial for maintaining the pH level of the culture medium, which is essential for embryonic development.

Tri-gas incubators: Tri-gas incubators are create an atmosphere with reduced oxygen levels, which is beneficial for the growth of embryos. Temperature and CO_2 concentration control in gas incubators are similar to those in CO_2 incubators. The desired oxygen concentration is achieved by injecting nitrogen gas into the chamber.

Time-lapse incubators: Time-lapse incubators have built-in camera imaging capabilities that allow monitoring and recording of embryonic development. This feature ensures observation of embryos throughout the developmental process.

Gas sensor calibration: Regularly calibrating the CO_2 and oxygen sensors using a calibrated gas mixture is a maintenance task that ensures that accurate and consistent measurements can be obtained by making reliable readings.

5.3.4 Microscopes

Stereomicroscopes, also known as dissecting microscopes, offer a three-dimensional view of samples. They have magnification capabilities typically ranging from 10× to 50×. These microscopes are especially useful for observing oocytes and embryos.

Inverted microscopes have an inverted path compared to upright microscopes. This means that the objective lens is positioned beneath the specimen stage, while the light source and eyepiece are located above it. This design allows for observation of cells and tissues in culture dishes during embryo assessment and micromanipulation procedures.

Phase contrast microscopy is a technique that enhances the visibility of specimens that may be difficult to see using bright field microscopy. By altering the phase of light passing through the specimen, this method improves visualisation.

Fluorescence microscopes utilise fluorescent markers attached to target molecules, which emit a glow when exposed to wavelengths of light. These microscopes are commonly used in ART labs for testing, research purposes, and imaging markers or structures within oocytes and embryos.

Compound microscopes are widely used in medicine and science fields. They offer versatility and are often favoured due to their ability to provide high-quality images across applications.

To obtain a magnified view of the sample, a sequence of lenses is used that results in an image. Compound microscopes are capable of observing specimens ranging from cells to bacteria to organisms.

5.3.5 Maintenance and Calibration

Cleaning the optics: The optical components of a microscope include lenses, mirrors, and other parts that aid in specimen viewing. It is important to keep these components clean and free from debris or smudges, as this directly affects image quality. A lint cloth or lens tissue along with a cleaning solution specifically designed for microscope optics should be used, while alcohol or harsh chemicals that could potentially damage the lens coatings should be avoided. The lenses should be handled delicately, without touching them with fingers or any other objects.

The illumination system of a microscope provides light for observing the specimen. The light source must be correctly positioned and adjusted to achieve the necessary brightness for imaging purposes. The mechanical elements of a microscope consist of the stage focus knobs and additional components that allow for movement and adjustment of the specimen. Regular inspections of these components are essential to ensure their operation and prevent any resistance. The stage must be level and stable, and the focus knobs must move smoothly without slipping or becoming stuck.

Calibrating the microscope: Calibration involves ensuring that the microscope produces measurements and images by adjusting the focus, aligning the optics, and verifying the magnification settings for accuracy.

5.3.6 Micromanipulation Systems

Micromanipulation systems are devices designed to precisely control and manipulate microtools. They enable procedures like intracytoplasmic sperm injection assisted hatching and embryo biopsy. These systems typically consist of three-axis control mechanisms (X, Y, and Z) that allow movements in all directions.

There are two types of micromanipulators.

Mechanical micromanipulators: These devices utilise gears, screws, and levers to achieve motion control. They often incorporate a fine-pitch screw that moves the tool a certain distance per rotation, such as 0.5 micrometres.

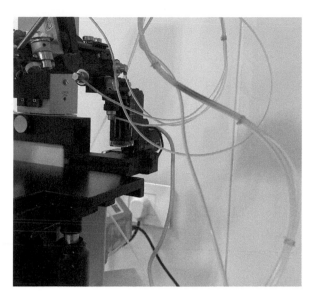

FIGURE 5.1
Photograph of micromanipulation tubing with blockage.

Hydraulic or pneumatic micromanipulators: These devices use oil or air pressure to regulate the motion of microtools. Manual valve controls aid in pressure adjustment, resulting in improved movement stability and smoothness. These systems employ closed-loop feedback control to maintain positioning and to counteract drift (Figure 5.1).

5.3.7 Microtools

Microinjectors: These tools typically feature a glass pipette with a tip. The diameter of the tip can range from 0.5 to 10 micrometres, depending on its intended purpose. This microinjector is connected to a pressure control system, which utilises either positive or negative pressure to regulate the flow of sperm during injection.

Microholders: These tools often employ vacuum pressure to securely hold cells, oocytes, or embryos in place. A vacuum pump generates the pressure, and its strength can be adjusted to prevent any harm to the oocyte or embryo.

Micropipettes: Similarly, micropipettes are crafted from glass pipettes that are hollow inside. They may feature tips that are bevelled for cell aspiration or biopsy purposes.

Calibration of micromanipulators: To ensure measurements, calibration is performed using a reference scale or stage micrometre with known dimensions. The micromanipulator is moved along the scale, and the distance travelled is compared against the expected distance based on the device's specifications.

Replacement of silicon sleeves: Some micromanipulators utilise silicon sleeves to create a surface and minimise contamination risks. It is important to replace these sleeves, as they may wear out over time.

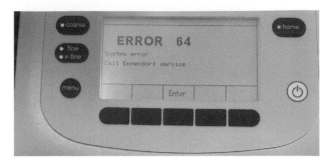

FIGURE 5.2
Photograph showing service error on the micromanipulator.

Maintenance of microinjectors: It is recommended to inspect the glass pipette of microinjectors for any signs of cracks or damage. Additionally, checking for clogging or debris that may impede the flow of injected substances at the tip is essential. Proper maintenance and cleaning of the pressure control system play a role in ensuring its operation (Figure 5.2).

5.3.8 Supporting Equipment

Microscopes: Inverted microscopes are commonly used for micromanipulation purposes, allowing for the visualisation of cells, oocytes, or embryos from below. To improve contrast and resolution compared to bright field microscopy, imaging techniques such as differential interference contrast (DIC) or Hoffman modulation contrast (HMC) are often employed.

Anti-vibration tables: These tables are designed to minimise vibrations using methods like mass, damping, and isolation techniques. They typically feature a top supported by air-filled bladders or mechanical springs that effectively absorb and dissipate vibrations originating from the surrounding environment.

Heating stages: Heating stages utilise Peltier elements to maintain a constant temperature during micromanipulation procedures. The temperature is accurately measured using either a thermocouple or a resistance temperature detector (RTD). A closed-loop feedback mechanism is then employed to regulate the temperature.

Software and computer systems: Micromanipulation systems come with software that offers real-time image processing capabilities along with automated data logging and statistical analysis. Depending on the complexity and purpose of the system, the software may provide complete automation of the micromanipulators' control. In systems, the integration of machine learning algorithms and computer vision methods can be utilised for tasks such as cell tracking, pattern identification, and decision-making during micromanipulation procedures.

5.3.9 Laser Systems

In ART labs, laser systems are utilised for procedures like assisted hatching and embryo biopsy. Assisted hatching involves using a laser to thin the zona pellucida, facilitating hatching and subsequent implantation.

There are two types of laser systems: Nd:YAG and diode lasers.

Operation: Neodymium doped yttrium aluminium garnet (Nd:YAG) lasers utilise a solid-state gain medium, a crystal infused with neodymium ions. The crystal is activated by either a flashlamp or diode laser to excite the neodymium ions into energy states. As these ions return to their energy state, they emit photons that stimulate the emission of photons, resulting in the creation of a coherent laser beam.

Wavelength: Nd:YAG lasers emit light at 1064 nm, falling within the infrared region of the spectrum. This wavelength's ability to be readily absorbed by water and its localised heating capabilities make it highly suitable for hatching procedures.

Pulse duration and energy: To create an opening in the zona pellucida, Nd:YAG lasers employ pulses of high-energy light typically ranging in the nanosecond scale (9–10 seconds).

The size and depth of the hole created during embryo biopsy can be controlled by adjusting the energy per pulse while also minimising harm to the embryo.

In contrast, diode lasers operate by generating a laser beam through indium gallium arsenide materials. By applying a current to these semiconductor materials, photons are created that create a coherent laser beam that can be used for embryo biopsy procedures.

Diode lasers typically operate at near-infrared wavelengths between 650 and 980 nm; this allows for controlled ablation of cells during biopsy while minimising damage to surrounding tissue.

When performing embryo biopsy procedures, it is common for lasers to have shorter pulse durations compared to Nd:YAG lasers. These pulse durations typically range from microseconds (6–10 seconds) to milliseconds (3–10 seconds), thus allowing for a controlled and gradual removal of cells. Additionally, the energy per pulse produced by lasers is lower than that of Nd:YAG lasers, reducing the risk of harm to the embryo.

They are generally smaller, lighter, and more affordable than Nd:YAG lasers, making them a favourable choice for IVF labs with budget limitations.

Diode lasers also offer flexibility in terms of wavelength emission, and they can be customised to emit wavelengths for different applications or to minimise damage to surrounding tissue.

5.3.10 Maintenance and Calibration

To ensure performance, regular maintenance and calibration are essential. It is important to inspect the laser system's lenses and mirrors for any dust, dirt, or damage. Cleaning should be done using a cloth or swab specifically designed for surfaces, along with an appropriate solvent formulated for such purposes.

Accurate alignment of the components plays a role in achieving the precise focus of the laser beam and ensuring optimal energy delivery to the intended target area.

The calibration process involves quantifying the energy or power of the laser beam using equipment like a laser power metre. Additionally, it entails adjusting the settings or components of the laser system to ensure that the measured energy or power falls within desired ranges. The goal is to align these measurements with established standards or reference values.

5.4 Cryopreservation Equipment

5.4.1 Understanding Liquid Nitrogen

One notable property of LN_2 is its boiling point of -196 °C (320 °F), because of which it is one of the substances most commonly employed in industrial and laboratory environments. This quality makes it particularly suitable for cryopreservation purposes.

Another interesting attribute is its expansion ratio. When LN_2 evaporates, it rapidly expands, with a volume expansion ratio of 1:694 (meaning that 1 litre of nitrogen produces roughly 694 litres of gaseous nitrogen). While this rapid expansion can be advantageous for applications, it requires management, as it can lead to pressure buildup in closed containers and can displace oxygen in confined spaces.

LN_2 does not readily react to other substances. This characteristic makes it an ideal choice in situations where chemical reactions need to be avoided. Another important aspect of LN_2 is that it is not flammable and does not support combustion. That said, while it is non-toxic, it can cause burns and frostbite upon contact with the skin or eyes due to its freezing temperature. A further advantage of LN_2 is its viscosity, which enables it to flow more rapidly compared to many other liquids. This property makes it convenient for transfer and manipulation within laboratory environments.

Liquid nitrogen also exhibits a high latent heat of vaporisation, meaning that when it transitions from a liquid to a gas state, it absorbs some heat energy. This characteristic renders it suitable as a coolant. Furthermore, nitrogen, which constitutes around 78% of the Earth's atmosphere, ensures the abundance and affordability of this resource.

5.4.2 Use of Liquid Nitrogen

The uses of LN_2 are incredibly versatile. It has applications in various sectors due to its unique characteristics, including its temperature, non-reactive properties, and significant expansion ratio.

One important use of LN_2 is cryopreservation, which is vital in research settings and which involves preserving sperm, eggs, embryos, tissues, and cells. LN_2 plays a role in procedures such as fertility treatments, stem cell studies, and conservation efforts for species.

In the field, liquid nitrogen is employed for cryosurgery to remove warts, skin tags, and certain types of skin cancer. The freezing temperature of LN_2 effectively destroys tissue while minimising damage to surrounding tissue.

Moreover, LN_2 serves as a coolant in the electronics industry during semiconductor and circuit manufacturing processes. By maintaining temperatures throughout production stages, LN_2 enhances efficiency and safeguards against damage.

Overall LN_2's adaptability makes it indispensable across industries. It finds application in the preservation of samples and materials through methods for long-term storage. The automotive and aerospace industries utilise LN_2 to test the performance and durability of materials and components at different temperatures. Moreover, for metalworking and welding purposes, LN_2 is utilised to shrink metal parts for assembly or disassembly. It also aids in cooling metals during machining processes, thereby reducing stress and distortion. Additionally, specific welding techniques benefit from LN_2 by minimising oxidation and improving weld quality.

In the chemical industry, LN_2 is employed to cool materials before grinding them into powders. This process prevents heat-sensitive substances from degrading while facilitating a grinding process. In rocket propulsion systems, LN_2 is occasionally used as a coolant for engine components. Its purpose is to maintain temperatures for proper engine functioning. Cryogenic storage tanks require the selection of insulation materials and temperature monitoring mechanisms.

5.4.3 Key Design Features of Cryostorage Tanks

Insulation: Cryostorage tanks use vacuum-insulated panels (VIPs) or perlite to minimise heat transfer and maintain low temperatures and therefore to preserve reproductive material.

Temperature monitoring: Manufacturers often incorporate temperature monitoring systems to ensure consistent temperatures. These systems include temperature sensors, thermocouples, or resistance temperature detectors. Connected to data loggers and alarm systems, these sensors help track and record temperature readings over time. The collected data is then analysed for monitoring purposes, while the alarm systems provide alerts if the temperature deviates from the desired range.

Cooling method: The choice of cooling method is crucial when designing cryostorage tanks. Each cooling method has its advantages and disadvantages, which depend on factors such as storage capacity, lab space, and safety considerations

Safety features: To prevent accidents and protect stored samples, cryostorage tanks are equipped with pressure relief valves, emergency shutoff valves, and oxygen monitors.

When designing cryostorage tanks, it is crucial to consider the design of the neck, which plays a role in minimising heat transfer and ensuring that ultra-low temperatures are maintained within the tank. The neck serves as the entrance and exit point for samples, allowing for insertion and retrieval.

Narrow diameter: To decrease heat transfer, the neck of a cryostorage tank is typically designed to have a narrow diameter; this reduces the surface area available for heat exchange.

Insulation: Insulation is also essential to achieving temperature control. Multiple layers of Mylar coated with either silver or aluminium are used to provide insulation. Additionally, incorporating vacuum-insulated walls in the neck area can further enhance insulation capabilities.

Tapered design: Some cryostorage tanks feature a neck design where the diameter gradually narrows towards the top. This design helps minimise the exposure of stored samples to air when the tank is opened, resulting in less heat entering the system.

Neck plug: When not in use, a removable neck plug or stopper is often employed to seal off the opening of the cryostorage tank. This plug fits securely within the tank neck, creating a barrier against exchange and maintaining extremely low temperatures.

Neck design and sample accessibility: The way the neck is designed and how easy it is to access samples stored in the cryostorage tank are interconnected. It is important to find a balance between minimising heat transfer and ensuring that samples can be easily inserted and retrieved when designing a plug that fits snugly within the neck. This can be achieved by using tools like canes or goblets and selecting a neck diameter that allows for access while also reducing heat entry into the system.

Maintenance: To maintain the desired temperature, it is crucial to check the nitrogen levels and refill as necessary. Additionally, the tanks must be inspected for any signs of damage or leaks, with prompt repairing or replacement when needed.

Cryovials: Cryovials are containers designed for storing samples at low temperatures. They are typically made from materials like polypropylene, a polycarbonate that can withstand cold conditions. Cryo-boxes are used to organise cryovials within the LN_2 storage tanks.

Maintenance: Cryovials should be regularly inspected for any indications of cracks, leaks, or compromised seals to prevent sample loss or contamination. Any damaged cryovials must be promptly replaced, and the cryo-boxes should be kept clean and well organised, with clear labelling for sample identification and retrieval.

Cryo-markers: For labelling cryovials and other equipment used in cryopreservation, specialised pens called cryo-markers are utilised. These markers are specially designed with ink that can withstand the temperatures of cryogenic storage as well as exposure to ethanol or isopropyl alcohol. Cryo-markers are created to endure low temperatures while still being readable. Using cryo-markers to label cryovials helps identify the content of each vial while ensuring the integrity of the samples.

Safety equipment: When dealing with materials at high temperatures during cryopreservation processes, it is recommended that individuals operating cryopreservation equipment wear cryogenic gloves, face shields, and aprons for their safety.

Maintenance: Safety equipment should be regularly inspected for any signs of wear or damage and replaced as necessary. Personnel should be properly trained on how to use and care for safety equipment to minimise the risks associated with handling materials.

Laboratory consumables: ART labs make use of pipettes, petri dishes, and other items. The quality of these consumables is crucial for the success of ART procedures.

Disposable pipettes: In ART labs, disposable pipettes are commonly used to handle and transfer embryos, gametes, and culture media. These pipettes are meant for one use only and should then be discarded.

Storage: Pipettes should be stored in their packaging in a clean and dry area away from direct sunlight or heat sources. It is crucial to check the packaging for any damage before using the pipette.

Petri dishes: These dishes are used for cultivating embryos and preparing culture media and other compounds. They are typically made of materials such as polystyrene or glass and come in various shapes and sizes (e.g., four wells, centre wells). For storage, it is recommended to keep them in their packaging in a clean and dry area.

5.4.4 Maintenance

Inventory management and the management of laboratory supplies are essential to maintaining their integrity. It is important to monitor inventory levels and pay attention to expiration dates to ensure the quality of stored products.

5.5 Equipment Logs

In ART laboratories, maintaining accurate equipment logs and implementing quality control measures are crucial for performance. Equipment logs help track equipment usage, maintenance, and calibration, while quality control measures aid in identifying and resolving issues.

By monitoring how this specialised equipment is utilised and its performance, lab personnel can detect problems and address them before they impact the results. Regulatory agencies may also request the maintenance of logs for equipment to demonstrate adherence to quality standards and guidelines.

For instance, if a lab uses laser systems for hatching or biopsy, they would keep a laser log to record the date, time, and relevant parameters for each laser use. Similarly, labs utilising micromanipulators for ICSI would maintain a micromanipulator log to document the date, time, type of needle used, and any observed issues during the procedure.

An incubator's comprehensive record should diligently note each temperature and CO_2 measurement checkup along with dates and times. It must also record any adjustments made to ensure embryo growth conditions as well as any irregularities detected during the incubation period.

The frequency of recording in specialised equipment logs may vary depending on the equipment used and procedures performed. To ensure the accuracy and completeness of the log, it is advisable to record any use of equipment in real time or immediately after the procedure. Laser systems or other equipment that is frequently used may require log entries, and it is crucial to keep them up to date for quality assurance and safety purposes.

When it comes to calibration and maintenance records, a standard calibration log should include details such as the calibration date, employed technique, and outcomes of the calibration process.

If any incidents or deviations occur while using the equipment, it is important to document them in the equipment log. For instance, if an alarm goes off on an incubator or LN_2 tank, it should be noted along with the actions taken to resolve the issue.

5.5.1 Importance of Equipment Logs

Many ART labs now rely on electronic equipment logs, which offer efficiency and lower chances of errors compared to paper logs. These electronic logs can be integrated with laboratory information management systems (LIMS) and provide real-time data on equipment performance and maintenance. Moreover, electronic logs provide automated alerts for calibrations or maintenance deadlines for added convenience.

The purpose of equipment logs is to ensure compliance by documenting performance and maintenance activities and to address any concerns regarding accuracy. During inspections, these logs play a role in demonstrating compliance and showcase a commitment to quality control. It is essential to maintain logs to track equipment during this procedure. These records provide information about the equipment's performance and maintenance, enabling lab staff to identify and address any issues that could affect lab results. Neglecting the maintenance of these records can have consequences such as loss of certification, penalties, and potential legal liability if a patient suffers harm or injury.

5.6 Preventive Maintenance Schedule

A preventive maintenance schedule (PMS) is a plan that outlines maintenance tasks performed on laboratory equipment to prevent breakdowns or malfunctions. An effective PMS plays a role in minimising breakdowns, optimising equipment performance, and ensuring compliance with standards.

Maintenance frequency: The frequency of maintenance activities depends on the type and usage of the equipment. For example, an incubator's PMS may include assessments of temperature and CO_2 levels, quarterly calibration, and the annual replacement of HEPA filters. Similarly, a microscope's PMS may involve cleaning and inspection of lenses and mechanical parts, quarterly calibration of magnification settings, and annual bulb replacement.

Documentation: It is essential to document all maintenance activities in the PMS. This documentation should include the date of maintenance, details about the type of maintenance performed, and any relevant notes regarding the condition of the equipment. Keeping a record like this helps track equipment performance over time, identify issues, and demonstrate compliance with regulatory requirements.

Integration with equipment logs: The PMS should be integrated with equipment logs to create a record of equipment performance and maintenance history. Equipment logs can capture any observed issues or abnormalities during maintenance activities.

5.6.1 Benefits of PMS

Enhanced safety: Checks and maintenance as part of a PMS significantly reduce the risk of accidents or hazardous situations. Engaging in this practice therefore plays a role in creating a safer working environment for laboratory personnel. Adhering to regulations and standards is an aspect of a PMS that supports ART labs. By following this approach, labs can ensure compliance with guidelines set by bodies like the FDA, WHO, or local authorities, thereby avoiding potential legal issues and penalties.

Moreover, adopting a maintenance routine significantly extends the lifespan of equipment by keeping it in optimal condition; this does not eliminate the need for premature replacement expenses but allows laboratories to maximise their investment.

In ART labs, where accuracy is paramount, regular maintenance of equipment is crucial. It actively contributes to upholding data accuracy by minimising the occurrence of results caused by equipment malfunctions.

Implementing a planned maintenance schedule brings benefits as well, enabling laboratories to make estimations regarding future costs while effectively budgeting for necessary maintenance and repairs. By adhering to a PMS, ART labs can act proactively and address equipment issues before they lead to downtime. This ensures that operations run smoothly without interruptions.

Having a maintenance system in place offers peace of mind to both staff members and management alike. They can rest assured knowing that the lab's equipment is diligently maintained and less prone to failure. Ultimately, implementing these practices leads to peak efficiency within ART labs by maintaining standards and safeguarding valuable resources.

Keeping equipment in good condition through maintenance is crucial, as it not only saves time during experiments and procedures but also improves productivity and reduces energy costs.

When it comes to customer satisfaction, equipment maintenance and calibration plays a significant role. It helps with fertilisation, embryo development, and cryopreservation, all of which ultimately contribute to treatment outcomes.

5.7 Model Log

In the laboratory, each piece of equipment should be distinctly identified by its model, serial number, and location. Every usage should be logged, noting the date, time, and user. Daily maintenance tasks, such as cleaning and calibration, must be detailed with respective dates and the person responsible. When malfunctions occur, all repairs or modifications should be documented, highlighting the date, individual in charge, and results. Calibration records ought to include dates, methods used, outcomes, and any necessary adjustments (Tables 5.1, 5.2, and 5.3).

TABLE 5.1

Sample 1: Equipment Logbook: MINC-Incubator

Equipment Identification	Installation Information	Calibration	Maintenance	Repairs	User Information	Signature
Equipment Name: Minc	Date of Installation:	Date of Last Calibration: 12/01/23	Date of Last Maintenance: 10/03/23	Date of Last Repair: Nil	Name of User: Smith	
Model Number: XYZ	Equipment Specifications: Trigas, Humidified	Calibration Results: Pass	Maintenance Performed By: John	Repair Details: Nil	Date/Time Used:	
Serial Number: 1234		Calibration Passed/ Failed:	Maintenance Performed:	Repair Performed by	Date/Time Used:	
Location: Embryology 1	Manufacturer's Manual: Yes	Next Calibration Due:	Next Maintenance Due:	Next Repair Due:	Date/Time Used:	
Comments/ Notes	Comments/ Notes:	Comments/ Notes:	Comments/ Notes:	Comments/ Notes:	Date/Time Used:	

TABLE 5.2

Sample 2: Equipment Logbook: Laminar Airflow

Equipment Identification	Installation Information	Calibration	Maintenance	Repairs	User Information	Signature
Equipment Name:	Date of Installation:	Date of Last Calibration:	Date of Last Maintenance:	Date of Last Repair:	Name of User:	
Model Number:	Installation Contraction:	Calibration Results:	Maintenance Performed By:	Repair Details:	Date/Time Used:	
Serial Number:	Equipment Specifications:	Calibration Passed/ Failed:	Maintenance Performed:	Repair Performed By:	Date/Time Used:	
Location:	Manufacturer's Manual:	Next Calibration Due:	Next Maintenance Due:	Next Repair Due:	Date/Time Used:	
Comments/ Notes:		Comments/ Notes:	Comments/ Notes:	Comments/ Notes:	Date/Time Used:	

TABLE 5.3

Sample 1: Preventive Maintenance Schedule

Equipment Name	Manufacturer	Model Number	Calibration Frequency	Maintenance Frequency	Next Calibration Due	Next Maintenance Due	Assigned To
Incubator-1	K-system	1234	Monthly	Quarterly	02/9/23	01/12/23	Mr Kennady
Incubator-1	Cook	5678	Monthly	Quarterly	05/09/23	04/12/23	Mr Kennady
Light Microscope	Olympus	1234	Monthly	Quarterly	03/09/23	04/12/23	Mr Kennady
Inverted Microscope	Nikon	5678	Monthly	Quarterly	03/09/23	04/12/23	Mr Kennady
Stereo zoom Microscope	Olympus	1234	Monthly	Quarterly	03/09/23	04/12/23	Mr Kennady
Laminar Airflow 1	IVF tech	12354	Monthly	Quarterly	08//09/23	07/12/23	Mr Kennady
Laminar Airflow 2	Clean Air	12345	Monthly	Quarterly	08/09/23	07/12/23	Mr Kennady
Micromanipulators	Eppendorf	22356	Monthly	Quarterly	09/09/23	08/12/23	Mr Kennady
Micromanipulators	Narishiage	56456	Monthly	Quarterly	09/09/23	08/12/23	Mr Kennady
Refrigerator	Samsung	4456	Monthly	Quarterly	12/09/23	11/12/23	Mr Kennady
Micropipettes	Eppendorf	54453	Quarterly	Quarterly	02/11/23	01/02/24	Mr John
CO_2 Analyser	Geo tech	4778	Quarterly	Quarterly	03/11/23	01/02/24	Mr John
pH meter	Hanah	8743	Quarterly	Quarterly	04/11/23	03/02/24	Mr John
Test tube warmer	Cook	4568	Quarterly	Quarterly	08/11/23	06/02/24	Mr John
Aspiration pump	Cook	41253	Quarterly	Quarterly	08/11/23	07/02/24	Mr John
Centrifuge	Eppendorf	45675	Quarterly	Quarterly	11/11/23	09/02/24	Mr John
Liquid nitrogen tank	Indian Oil	54645		Monthly		04/02/24	Mr John

CHAPTER 5

SUMMARY

- The optimal performance and prevention of equipment failure are contingent upon each equipment type's appropriate maintenance and calibration.
- Quality control assessments on lab consumables, such as pipettes, culture dishes, and media, are critical to ensuring accurate and reliable results.
- Avoiding contamination requires adhering to strict procedures for managing, storing, and disposing of consumables.
- Equipment logs should include the date, technician name, tasks executed, and any identified issues.
- ART labs must maintain a preventive maintenance schedule to reduce equipment downtime and prevent failure.
- The execution of preventive maintenance tasks requires the cleaning, calibration, and replacement of parts as required.
- A preventive maintenance schedule helps equipment perform better and prevents costly repairs and downtime.
- ART laboratories guarantee a secure and safe environment for ART procedures by adhering to strict equipment maintenance and calibration guidelines.
- Proper equipment maintenance and calibration help with adequate fertilisation, embryo development, and cryopreservation, ultimately contributing to successful treatment outcomes and patient satisfaction.

6

Quality Control of ART Media and Disposables

In ART laboratories, a range of culture media is commonly utilised because of their high-quality, consistent properties and user friendliness. These media offer the essential nutrients and ideal environments for the in vitro growth and evolution of embryos. Typically, these media consist of amino acids, vitamins, minerals, and other essential nutrients required for embryonic growth. Additionally, they may also contain growth factors and hormones to support stages of embryonic development. The design objective is to mimic the environment found in the fallopian tube so that embryos can thrive and develop outside the human body.

6.1 Media for Handling Gametes

Human tubal fluid (HTF): HTF is formulated to replicate the environment found in the tubes. It is isotonic and buffered with N-2-hydroxyethylpiperazine-N'-2-ethanesulfonic acid (HEPES) or bicarbonate to maintain pH levels. HTF contains glucose, pyruvate, amino acids, and albumin—all components that support gamete survival and functioning.

Sperm washing media: Sperm washing media is specifically designed to separate motile sperm from plasma, debris, and non-motile sperm. These media contain components that help preserve sperm viability and motility, such as HEPES buffer.

6.2 Oocyte Maturation

In vitro maturation (IVM) media: For the oocyte to function optimally, it requires calcium, magnesium, and zinc, as well as specific amino acids such as L-glutamine and L-alanine. FSH and LH play a role in resuming meiosis and breaking down the vesicle, while epidermal growth factor (EGF) supports the expansion of cumulus cells, which is crucial for oocyte maturation. These media may also include cysteine and glutathione to provide protection against stress.

Single-step media: Monophasic media, also known as single-step media, are created with a balance of nutrients, growth factors, and hormones to facilitate embryonic growth from fertilisation until blastocyst formation without requiring any changes in the media used. The continuous culture method incorporates elements that serve as energy sources, such as non-essential amino acids, glucose, pyruvate, and lactate. Growth factors like EGF and transforming growth factor-beta (TGF β)

DOI: 10.1201/9781032622736-6

as well as hormones like insulin and insulin-like growth factor (IGF) are included to support growth. Collectively, these components create an environment that facilitates development.

Sequential media: Sequential media formulations are specifically designed for stages of embryo development.

Usually, in the initial three days of embryo culture, the media might include amino acids and glucose. But from days 4 to 6, the media might also have these elements in higher concentrations, complemented by growth factors. This assists the transition from the cleavage phase to the blastocyst stage.

For fertilisation, specific media are used that are supplemented with calcium, potassium, and sodium ions. These ions help maintain balance and support sperm capacitation. The media also include bicarbonate and HEPES buffers for pH control. Albumin plays a role in removing reactive oxygen species (ROS) and providing fatty acids. Additionally, hyaluronan supports sperm motility and stability.

During the cleavage stage, specialised media are used that contain L-arginine, L-lysine, and L-glutamine. These components aid in protein synthesis and embryo development. The media also provide glucose, pyruvate, vitamins, and minerals for functioning. Regarding blastocyst culture, specific media are employed that have a proportion of non-essential amino acids. This is necessary to support increased protein synthesis during this phase. Additionally, these media can be enriched with growth factors such as EGF or TGF β to promote inner cell mass (ICM) and trophoblast progression.

6.3 Micromanipulation Media

G MOPS (Gentle MOPS): It contains MOPS (3 [N morpholino] propane acid), a buffer that maintains the pH of the medium within a range. G MOPS is designed for short-term use during procedures like oocyte retrieval, denudation, and ICSI. However, it is not suitable for long-term culturing or the incubation of embryos.

Polyvinylpyrrolidone (PVP): PVP is a substance that helps regulate sperm motility during ICSI. It acts as a neutral polymer that attaches to the sperm membrane, preventing capacitation and increasing the chances of fertilisation.

Hyaluronidase: Hyaluronidase is an enzyme; it is naturally present in the oophorus, which forms a layer around the oocyte. In ART, hyaluronidase is commonly used to remove this layer by dissolving its hyaluronic acid structure. This process frees the oocyte from surrounding cumulus cells. This particular step plays a role in evaluating the maturity of the oocyte and preparing it for procedures such as ICSI.

Freezing media: Vitrification is a method of freezing that involves different concentrations of cryoprotectants and ultra-rapid cooling rates, typically achieved through liquid nitrogen. The vitrification solution contains levels (up to 40%) of ethylene glycol, DMSO, and sucrose, which protect the cells from ice crystal formation during the cooling process.

Thawing media: Thawing solutions safely bring cryopreserved cells to room temperature for use in ART procedures. Thawing solutions usually contain high concentrations of cryoprotectants that restore the cell's natural environment, balance pressure, and prevent cellular damage during thawing.

6.4 Storage of IVF Media

It is critical to store IVF media within an optimal temperature range to ensure their stability and effectiveness, with most culture media typically requiring a range between 2–8 °C. Furthermore, protection from light exposure is equally important; hence, many containers used for ART lab media are designed to be opaque or are treated with coatings that block out light (Figure 6.1).

Shelf life: IVF media have a shelf life, meaning they can only be stored for a certain period before they expire. The actual shelf life may vary depending on the composition and manufacturer.

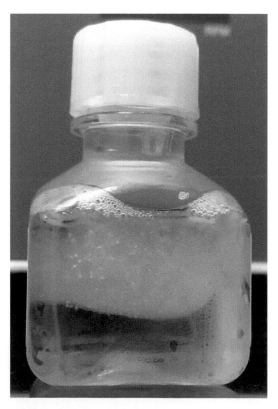

FIGURE 6.1
Photograph showing IVF medium in a frozen state.

6.5 Types of Quality Control Tests for IVF Media

Quality control plays a role in ensuring the viability of embryos or gametes when using IVF media. As part of quality control measures, multiple tests are carried out to ensure that embryos, oocytes, and spermatozoa used in ART procedures are free from any contamination that could potentially pose risks.

Sterility testing: There are multiple methods for sterility testing, such as direct inoculation, membrane filtration, and the most probable number (MPN) method.

- In the inoculation technique, a small amount of the sample is added to a medium.
- Membrane filtration involves passing a known volume of the media or reagent through a filter with defined size. This filter retains any microorganisms in the sample. The retained membrane is then transferred to a medium.
- The MPN method includes diluting the media or reagent and introducing it into a medium. The number of negative test results is then used to calculate the probable number of microorganisms present.

Endotoxin testing: Endotoxins are substances composed of lipopolysaccharides found in the cell walls of gram-negative bacteria. A common method for performing this testing is by using the Limulus amebocyte lysate (LAL) assay. This approach utilises a reagent derived from the horseshoe crab. The reagent contains an enzyme that reacts uniquely with endotoxins resulting in the formation of a gel. The more gel that forms, the greater the concentration of endotoxins in the tested sample.

pH testing: The pH level of IVF media should be maintained between 7.2 and 7.4 to ensure embryos' growth and development; this can be measured using either a pH metre or pH indicator strips that assess the hydrogen ion concentration in the sample.

Osmolality testing: An osmometer is used to measure the solute concentration in the sample. The utilised method for measuring osmolality involves freezing point depression, which determines the decrease in freezing point caused by solute presence.

Performance testing: During these tests, we culture embryos in the media and carefully observe their growth and development. Our goal is to ensure that the media effectively support the embryos growth and development, resulting in high-quality embryos that can be safely transferred or preserved through cryopreservation.

Stability testing: To assess the stability of our media and reagents, we subject them to temperature and humidity level tests. This helps us determine how well they resist varying conditions. During stability testing, we store the media for a period of time, then evaluate their quality through control tests to ensure performance and reliability, guaranteeing that they continue to meet their intended use and specifications over time.

6.6 Overseeing the QC of an Open IVF Media Pack

Opened media packs in an IVF laboratory require more attention compared to sealed ones due to the increased risk of exposure to potential contaminants. Since the entire pack may not be used immediately, it becomes necessary to store it. However, this storage introduces risks such as air exposure, light intrusion, temperature fluctuations, and potential contamination. These factors can have an impact on the quality and consistency of the IVF media. Therefore, it is extremely important to follow manufacturer guidelines and SOPs for handling and storing these opened packs from a quality control perspective. The following steps must be followed.

- Attach a label indicating the date and time of opening to keep track of the pack's usage.
- Store packs of IVF media in a controlled environment, maintaining a temperature of 2–8 °C and a humidity of 50%–70%. Regularly monitor temperature and humidity levels, discarding any media that have been contaminated or that have expired.
- Close IVF media packs when not in use to prevent evaporation. Contamination can introduce bacteria, fungi, or other microorganisms that may affect embryonic development. Store the pack in a dry place for preservation.
- Adhere to the manufacturer's instructions when determining the recommended duration for using packs of IVF media. After this designated period has passed, it is necessary to dispose the bottle.
- It is advisable to check the pH and osmolality of open-pack media as part of quality control measures. Detecting any changes promptly will help maintain quality and effectiveness while avoiding negative effects on patients.
- Using a laminar flow hood and following media preparation techniques can help prevent contamination.
- To avoid cross-contamination, it is important not to use packs of media simultaneously. It is recommended that each pack be used for a procedure, and all equipment should be carefully cleaned and sterilised after each use to minimise hazards.
- Before using any media, make sure to check the expiration date and discard any expired ones.

QC documentation: This documentation should include details such as the name of the media, batch number, manufacturing date, ingredients used, manufacturing procedure followed, test results obtained, and expiration date. This information helps identify and address any issues with the media before it is used.

- Quality control documentation plays a role in enhancing the quality of media, minimising the risk of contamination, increasing lab efficiency, and ensuring compliance with standards.

The following points offer examples of how quality control documentation is utilised to enhance the safety and effectiveness of ART lab media.

- Documenting test results helps verify that the media meets all required standards.
- Keeping track of expiration dates prevents the use of expired media, which could pose risks to patients' well-being.
- Certificates of analysis (CoAs) provide a summary of testing results for each batch of media to confirm its adherence to specifications. CoAs typically cover aspects such as sterility, endotoxin levels, pH balance, osmolality, and mouse embryo assay (MEA) outcomes.
- Product specifications offer a breakdown of the composition and characteristics of the media. This includes information about component concentrations, pH levels, osmolality, ionic strength, storage requirements, and shelf life.
- Bacterial endotoxin tests are typically carried out using the LAL test, with results that must be below the specified limit (0.25 EU/mL).
- MEA testing is widely applied during preparation to ascertain the media's efficacy in supporting embryo development. The MEA acts as a benchmark to ensure the quality of both the media and the materials used in ART.
- Stability testing conducted under controlled storage conditions provides information about the shelf life of the media. Expiration dates and appropriate storage conditions (e.g., 28 °C, protected from light) are clearly indicated.
- Traceability records involve assigning a lot number to each batch of media. These records help to quickly identify any batches for removal from use in cases of contamination or performance issues. By tracking the lot numbers used in each procedure, embryologists can monitor how well the media performs over time, identify patterns in outcomes, and make protocol adjustments.

To ensure the handling, storage, and testing of these materials, it is crucial to follow the recommended protocols and manufacturer instructions and maintain thorough documentation. This diligent approach plays a role in preserving the effectiveness and viability of these resources for patients undergoing fertility treatments.

CHAPTER 6

SUMMARY

- Appropriate quality control measures are mandatory to ensure the efficacy and safety of the used media.
- Testing IVF media involves sterility, endotoxin levels, pH, osmolality, and visual inspection. It ensures that the media are safe and effective for IVF procedures, ultimately enhancing the chances of successful implantation and pregnancy.
- The purpose of conducting these tests is to verify the absence of any potential contaminants, confirm all required chemical properties, and establish the safety of the media for use in ART procedures.

- Maintaining the integrity of IVF media requires adherence to appropriate storage conditions.

- Regular monitoring of storage conditions is required to ensure the viability of the media.

- IVF media is a complex mixture of nutrients and other substances essential for embryo growth and development. Once opened, the media begins to degrade, and its effectiveness declines over time. Therefore, it is vital to use IVF media within the recommended timeframe and to discard any unused media.

- The recommended timeframe for IVF media varies depending on the specific media and the manufacturer's instructions.

- QC testing for IVF media must be well documented to provide responsibility and traceability.

- Records of quality control tests must contain the date, test results, and the name of the technician who carried out the test.

- This document thoroughly outlines the media's composition, providing specifics on the concentrations of all components, the pH value, osmolality, and ionic strength.

- Adhering to stringent quality control standards for IVF media and disposable materials is crucial to ensure a reliable and secure setting for assisted reproduction. Compliance with these standards ensures they meet requirements and specifications, thus mitigating potential risks and maximising the success of the procedures.

7

IVF Process and QC

In the health field, it is crucial for laboratories specialising in fertility assessments to obtain reliable results. Having a grasp of the IVF process enables ART laboratory staff to implement quality control measures at every stage of the procedure. It is essential to have an understanding of each step, from stimulation to embryo transfer, as they require specific conditions and meticulous handling. Furthermore, embryologists play a role in establishing and monitoring quality control procedures to maintain standards in their lab practices (Figure 7.1).

7.1 QC in Andrology

7.1.1 Overview of Standard Andrology Lab Procedures

7.1.1.1 Semen Analysis

Semen analysis is a step in assessing male fertility. This evaluation involves measuring parameters such as volume, sperm count, motility, morphology, and the presence of cells like leukocytes. Low sperm counts and poor motility are often linked to infertility. Sperm motility refers to the ability of sperm to move forward effectively. Additionally, abnormal structure or shape of the sperm can hinder ability to fertilise an egg.

7.2 QC in CASA

Automated systems for sperm analysis utilise imaging technologies and computer vision algorithms to quantitatively analyse sperm samples. These sophisticated systems efficiently examine thousands of sperm cells, providing data on factors such as sperm count, motility, morphology, and DNA fragmentation. Moreover, laboratories that utilise automated sperm analysis setups must adhere to calibration, maintenance, and proficiency examination protocols to ensure the accuracy of the results.

7.3 Standard Semen Preparation Techniques

Swim-up technique: The swim-up technique is commonly chosen as the method for selecting motile sperm for ART. This approach operates on the principle that energetically swimming sperm move from the plasma into a culture medium.

DOI: 10.1201/9781032622736-7

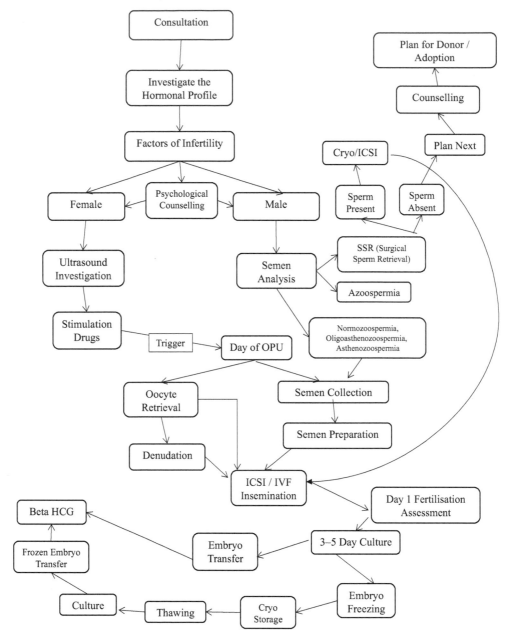

FIGURE 7.1
Schematic overview of the IVF process.

Density gradient centrifugation: In this method, the semen sample is layered on top of a two-tiered gradient and then centrifuged. The motile and morphologically normal sperm migrate through the gradient and accumulate at the bottom of the tube, while non-motile sperm, debris, and other cells remain in the layers.

Microfluidic devices: Microfluidic devices are an addition to the array of techniques used for sperm preparation. These methods contribute to enhancing understanding of fertility by enabling assessments in ART laboratories.

These devices utilise channels and compartments to separate active sperm from inactive sperm and unwanted particles via motion and size. Microfluidic devices typically operate with small amounts of semen and have the ability to produce a highly refined sample of sperm.

Sperm freezing and thawing: Sperm freezing is especially beneficial for patients who may need treatment cycles or who are at risk due to treatments that can affect fertility. Thawing refers to the process of warming the sperm to make them viable again for use in IVF. To ensure quality control, proper labelling and storage of samples, monitoring temperature changes during thawing, and evaluating thawing motility and viability are important steps.

Assessing sperm DNA fragmentation: Elevated levels of DNA fragmentation can hinder conception. The sperm chromatin structure assay (SCSA) is a method used to examine DNA integrity. It involves using Acridine Orange, a dye that distinguishes between sperm with intact DNA and those with damaged DNA. Another technique used to evaluate sperm DNA integrity is the TUNEL (terminal deoxynucleotidyl transferase dUTP nick end labelling) assay. This method detects fragmented DNA by incorporating labelled nucleotides at the break sites.

The comet assay, or single-cell gel electrophoresis, is also employed to assess sperm DNA fragmentation levels. In this process, cells are placed in a gel on a microscope slide and exposed to electrophoresis, which employs a field to separate molecules. When DNA is damaged, it migrates further in the gel, creating a comet 'tail' that gives the assay its name. The length and intensity of this tail indicate the extent of DNA damage. Understanding levels of sperm DNA fragmentation helps clinicians customise treatment plans for individuals based on their needs.

7.4 Surgical Sperm Aspiration

In cases of azoospermia, techniques like testicular sperm extraction (TESE) and microsurgical epididymal sperm aspiration (MESA) are useful, as they allow retrieval of sperm from the epididymis.

7.5 Quality Control

- Quality control plays a role in andrology laboratories, as it ensures accuracy, reproducibility, and reliability in procedures while prioritising safety and effectiveness.
- To maintain accurate outcomes in andrology procedures, it is crucial to establish SOPs and adhere to them.
- Regular equipment maintenance and calibration are important aspects. Calibration involves using reference materials with known properties to check measurements. It is necessary to maintain calibration certificates or records for each instrument that document the calibration date, reference standards used, and obtained results.

- Method validation and verification are steps that ensure the reliability and credibility of procedures in andrology labs.
- Andrology validation is a process that ensures the accuracy, precision, sensitivity, specificity, and robustness of a test method before it is implemented. It involves assessing analytical performance characteristics, establishing reference ranges, and evaluating any limitations. Verification is carried out when introducing a method or making changes to an existing one. It ensures that the method functions as intended within the laboratory setting and confirms its reliability for diagnostic purposes.
- Quality assurance and quality improvement programmes play a role in maintaining standards. Internal quality control enables laboratories to monitor their performance by using control materials to identify any errors or inconsistencies. External quality assessment programmes provide an evaluation of laboratory performance by comparing results with reference values and other participating laboratories.
- Documentation and record-keeping are important aspects of andrology procedures. Thorough documentation supports traceability, simplifies troubleshooting processes, and acts as a resource during audits to ensure compliance.

7.6 Troubleshooting

Sperm preparation issues: Troubleshooting issues may arise during sperm preparation. Problems could occur during swim-up or during density gradient processes for sperm samples. In some cases, adjusting the protocol or modifying parameters like duration speed can potentially improve outcomes.

If there are problems, it might be worth exploring alternative methods of sperm preparation (Figure 7.2).

Challenges in procedures for retrieving sperm: Procedures like TESE can sometimes encounter difficulties in obtaining a suitable amount of sperm.

7.7 Solution

Making adjustments to the approach or utilising tools and microsurgical techniques could potentially improve the success rate of sperm retrieval.

When exploring retrieval techniques, if initial attempts are unsuccessful, it may be beneficial to consider methods like microdissection TESE (micro TESE) or percutaneous epididymal sperm aspiration (PESA).

Exploring options: Offering support and guidance to patients regarding alternative fertility options such as donor sperm or adoption can be crucial in cases where retrieval is not possible.

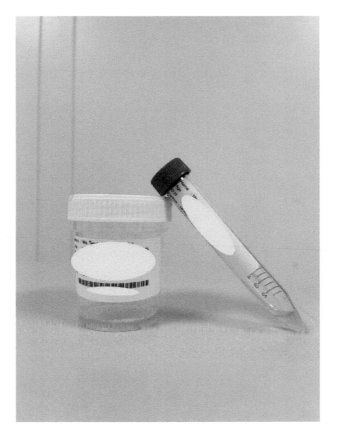

FIGURE 7.2
Photograph showing labelling process of semen preparation.

Equipment issues: Regular maintenance and a comprehensive schedule for upkeep of laboratory equipment, coupled with consistent calibration and quality control measures, ensure optimal performance and reliable and precise results while promptly addressing malfunctioning equipment through timely repairs or replacements and guarantee seamless operation in the andrology laboratory.

Human errors: Incorrect specimen labelling or procedural inaccuracies can occur in andrology laboratories. Occasionally, procedural errors may happen in andrology laboratories.

7.8 Troubleshooting of Human Error

Human error can be avoided through a combination of training and ongoing education for laboratory staff to improve their skills and understanding of procedures. Regular quality control inspections should also be conducted to identify any errors and allow for corrections to adhere to established protocols and best practices.

By addressing troubleshooting scenarios in andrology procedures, professionals can successfully overcome challenges, thereby guaranteeing the provision of precise and dependable results.

CHAPTER 7

SUMMARY

- Andrology is essential to ART laboratories, focusing on male fertility and related procedures.
- Semen analysis is a basic andrology procedure that assesses sperm concentration, motility, and morphology.
- Swim-up, density gradient centrifugation, and simple wash are employed to isolate high-quality sperm and increase the likelihood of successful fertilisation.
- Quality control in andrology is crucial for ensuring the accuracy and reliability of laboratory results and maintaining a high standard of patient care.
- Troubleshooting common andrology procedure problems involves addressing low sperm count, poor motility, abnormal morphology, and contamination.
- Regular maintenance and calibration of equipment and staff training are essential to minimise errors and ensure smooth laboratory operations.
- Following established protocols and guidelines provided by the World Health Organisation is essential to enhancing the quality of andrology services in ART laboratories.
- Continuous monitoring and evaluation of laboratory processes and procedures are necessary to identify areas of improvement and to maintain high success rates in ART.
- Effective communication among laboratory staff and collaboration with other healthcare professionals can help optimise patient outcomes and laboratory performance.
- Advancements in technology and research will continue to shape andrology practices, leading to improved diagnostic and treatment options for male infertility.

8

Quality Control in Embryo Culture

It is important to ensure that the process of culturing embryos is done well to achieve successful outcomes in ART. Embryo culturing goes through quality control procedures that involve technological methods and strict protocols. These measures are in place to promote embryo development. The most viable embryos are then selected for transfer. Quality control in embryo culture can be broadly categorised into two interconnected components: laboratory quality control and embryo quality control.

8.1 Embryo Culture Conditions

The conditions of culturing embryos in a lab setting are crucial for their growth. To create the environment, a formulated medium is used that contains a combination of salts, glucose, amino acids, and essential nutrients. It is important to control the pH level of the medium to ensure embryo development. Incubators play a role in maintaining conditions such as temperature, humidity, and gas levels to effectively support the embryo's growth (Figure 8.1).

8.2 Monitoring Embryo Development

Morphological assessment: Assessments of the embryo's morphology are subjective and depend on the skill of the embryologist. However, this challenge can be overcome by implementing monitoring and utilising objective criteria for selecting embryos with the assistance of time-lapse technology (Figure 8.2).

Typically, when evaluating embryos, we consider factors like cell number, symmetry, fragmentation, and the presence of cells. Embryos that have a cell count corresponding to their stage and that exhibit symmetrical characteristics are generally regarded as having good potential for viability. On the other hand, fragmentation indicates compromised quality, while multinucleated cells suggest issues with cell division and inferior embryonic quality.

During day 1 (16–18 hours after insemination), successful fertilisation is confirmed by observing two pronuclei. On days 2 and 3 (cleavage stage), assessments are made regarding cell number, symmetry, and fragmentation.

As embryos progress to the blastocyst stage, their evaluation is based on their expansion level and the appearance of the inner cell mass (ICM) and trophectoderm (TE) layers.

DOI: 10.1201/9781032622736-8

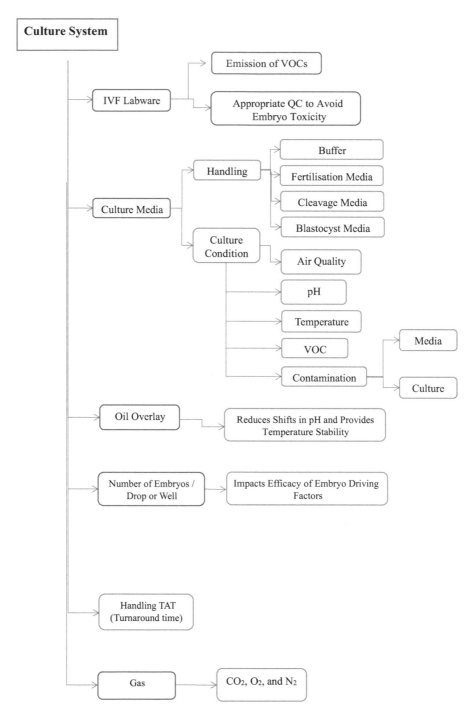

FIGURE 8.1
Schematic flowchart of embryo culture system.

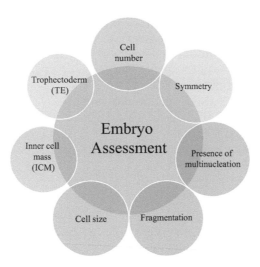

FIGURE 8.2
Factors influencing embryo assessment.

The Gardner grading system is commonly used to evaluate the quality of blastocysts in ART. It involves assigning a grade ranging from 1 to 6 that considers factors such as expansion level, ICM quality (graded as A, B, or C), and TE quality (also graded as A, B, or C). This grading system helps classify embryos in ART procedures.

8.3 Timelapse Imaging

Timelapse imaging technology is a tool for embryologists to observe and monitor changes in embryos without causing any disturbance to their incubator environment. By analysing the development patterns and detecting any irregularities or delays in growth through these timelapse images, embryologists can select embryos for transfer, which ultimately increases the chances of a successful outcome. However, it is important to note that there may be variations in grading systems among embryologists due to individual subjectivity.

Another significant technique, preimplantation genetic testing (PGT), involves examining the composition of embryos to gain insights into their genetic health. This process includes extracting two to four trophectoderm cells from each embryo and subjecting them to analysis.

8.4 Metabolomic Profiling

Profiling is an approach that focuses on analysing metabolites, or molecules produced by cells during their metabolic processes. When applied to evaluating embryo quality, this method involves studying the culture medium. As an embryo develops, it interacts with its environment by absorbing nutrients from the culture medium and releasing metabolites into it. These metabolites encompass amino acids, proteins, sugars, and lipids; they essentially represent the end products of reactions within the embryo. By examining the presence, absence, or amounts of these metabolites, we can gain insights into an embryo's metabolic health and potential.

Metabolomic profiling in culture media allows embryologists to assess alterations in composition without procedures. This assessment helps inform decisions regarding the selection of embryos for transfer or cryopreservation. Notably, while metabolomic profiling holds promise, ongoing research and development are still exploring its practicality and usefulness in real-world applications.

> **Artificial intelligence (AI):** Embryo assessment in ART has traditionally relied on the repetitive observation of embryos under a microscope throughout various stages of their development. However, this approach can be laborious, time consuming, and somewhat subjective, as it heavily relies on the experience and judgement of the embryologist.

By leveraging algorithms, AI and machine learning (ML) technologies introduce objectivity and standardisation to embryo assessment. They eliminate variability by analysing the parameters of embryos more accurately and efficiently. The combination of AI and ML with time-lapse imaging techniques is particularly beneficial in handling large volumes of data related to embryonic development. This type of imaging generates data that can be challenging to analyse. However, AI and ML efficiently process this data, identifying patterns and characteristics associated with embryonic development that may not be noticeable to observers.

Additionally, AI and ML models have the ability to continuously learn and improve their accuracy over time by analysing accumulated data. This self-improvement aspect proves advantageous in enhancing the precision of the embryo selection process with each cycle.

However, it is important to recognise that the integration of AI and ML in ART is still in its early stages. While these technologies hold promise, further adoption and optimisation are necessary. Ongoing research and development efforts are focused on improving the performance and accessibility of AI and ML tools while also addressing regulatory considerations.

> **Embryo transfer:** Before embryo transfer, it is important to conduct an evaluation of the patient's medical history, the condition of their uterus, and the receptivity of their endometrium. This evaluation includes assessing and documenting factors like any issues with the uterus (like fibroids or polyps) as well as the thickness and appearance of the endometrium. It is crucial to identify and address any problems that could affect implantation, such as adhesions or chronic inflammation in the uterus.

It is crucial to follow techniques such as maintaining hand hygiene, using draping and equipment to prevent contamination, and reducing the chances of infections. Selecting the catheter for embryo transfer is of importance. It is crucial to take into account factors such as the traits of the patient, their experiences with transfers, and the expertise provided by embryologists. When using ultrasound guidance during the transfer process, it provides a representation of where the catheter tip is positioned inside the uterus cavity. To ensure placement and minimise any complications associated with catheter usage, it is crucial to adhere to the guidance provided by ultrasound imaging. After the embryo transfer

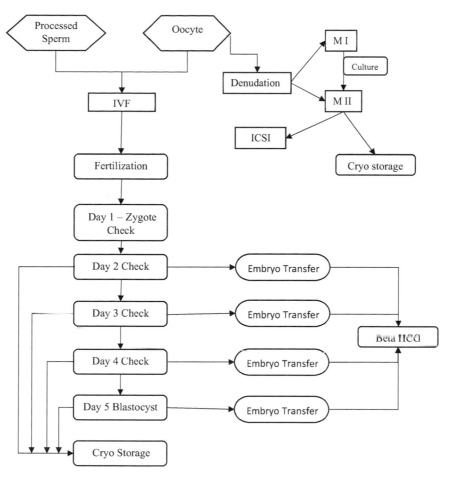

FIGURE 8.3
Flowchart of steps leading to successful embryo transfer.

providing transfer care and regular follow-up is crucial for a successful implantation. It is also necessary to prescribe and administer medications like progesterone supplementation based on established protocols, scheduling follow-up appointments to monitor progress and evaluate implantation (Figure 8.3).

By highlighting correct procedures along with the significance of quality control measures, embryologists can contribute to achieving safe embryo transfer procedures in ART laboratories. Adhering to protocols, ensuring selection and verification of equipment, and providing comprehensive patient care are vital steps in attaining positive outcomes in ART procedures.

8.5 Troubleshooting Embryo Culture Problems

There are factors that can contribute to issues in embryo culture, including the composition of the culture media, incubator conditions, laboratory practices, and environmental factors. When troubleshooting these problems, it is important to take a comprehensive approach that considers all sources of variation and error.

These steps can be followed to address any issues.

Check the culture medium: Review the expiration date, storage conditions, and batch number of the medium used. Select a medium that matches the stage of embryonic development.

Evaluate the pH of the culture medium: The ideal pH for optimal embryonic development is between 7.2–7.4. Factors such as the composition of the gas atmosphere and the sealing of the culture dish can affect pH levels.

Inspect culture dishes and microtools: Look at the quality and sterility of culture dishes, pipettes, and other microtools used in embryo manipulation. Always use certified plasticware that is non-toxic, and ensure cleaning and sterilisation before use.

Exposure: Prolonged exposure to ultraviolet light can have negative effects on embryonic development. Limit embryos exposure to light as much as possible during manipulations. Use low-intensity illumination when needed.

Review handling techniques: Ensure that all laboratory personnel are well trained in embryo handling techniques to avoid temperature fluctuations or unnecessary manipulations during procedures. Assess lab workflow to minimise how long embryos are kept outside of incubators.

Ensure the quality of sperm and eggs: Assess the quality of gametes to avoid compromised embryos. Use quality sperm and eggs by evaluating preparation and selection techniques for fertilisation.

Prevent contamination: Contamination from bacteria or fungi can harm embryonic development. Maintain a sterile environment by sanitising work surfaces, equipment, and incubators. Follow techniques and sterile handling procedures to minimise the risk of contamination.

Monitor air quality in the laboratory: The presence of VOCs and particulate matter in the lab environment can impact embryonic development. Regularly check that air filtration systems are functioning optimally through air quality assessments.

Evaluate staff expertise: Assess the proficiency of laboratory personnel to maintain standards in an ART lab. All staff members should be well trained and experienced in IVF techniques, as human error can contribute to problems during embryo culturing, potentially affecting treatment outcomes.

Follow cryopreservation and thawing protocols: Freezing and thawing embryos require adherence to established protocols. Proper handling is essential for improving embryo survival rates.

Train personnel on embryo assessment: Provide training on techniques for assessing and grading embryos. Accurate evaluation helps identify issues guiding decision-making throughout the ART process.

Designing and organising a laboratory: Optimise the design and layout of a laboratory to promote smooth workflows and minimise the risk of contamination. To prevent any possibility of cross-contamination, it is recommended to maintain separate areas for oocyte retrieval, embryo handling, and cryopreservation.

Quality management system: Implementing a quality management system (QMS) ensures that an ART laboratory consistently provides high-quality care for patients.

Consideration of external factors: Consider the impact of external factors, such as stress, on individuals undergoing ART treatment.

Audits and inspections: Establish a schedule for conducting both internal and external audits; this helps to evaluate laboratory procedures and identify areas for improvement as well as ensures compliance with standards and regulations.

8.6 Issue 1: Poor Embryo Quality

- Make adjustments to the culture conditions, such as pH levels, osmolality, or gas concentrations, to create an environment that closely mimics nature.
- Enhance laboratory techniques by minimising embryo handling and reducing exposure to factors like light, temperature fluctuations, or vibrations.
- It is important to note that the effective solution when addressing embryo quality depends on individual factors and the underlying cause of the issue.

8.7 Issue 2: Embryo Growth

- Fine-tune culture conditions by adjusting temperature and CO_2 levels.
- Consider changing to a type of media that better supports embryo growth.
- Delaying embryo transfer until reaching the blastocyst stage might improve chances of implantation for embryos experiencing growth.

8.8 Issue 3: Embryo Arrest

- Making adjustments to the conditions, such as pH levels, oxygen levels, and nutrient availability, can positively impact embryo development. Optimising these factors increases the chances of growth and development.
- Continuous monitoring of embryos through timelapse imaging enables detection of any irregularities or delays in their growth. This valuable information allows for adjustments in culture conditions or other interventions if required.
- To closely monitor embryo growth and identify any abnormalities or delays, it is beneficial to incorporate timelapse imaging into the process.
- Enhancing embryo development can involve using quality culture media or changing the type of media used.
- Minimising exposure to light, temperature fluctuations and vibrations during development can also contribute to successful outcomes.

8.9 Issue 4: Fluctuations in Success Rates

- Fluctuations in success rates can occur due to various factors, such as differences in how the laboratory operates, changes in the types of patients treated, and external influences on outcomes.
- To address this issue, ART laboratories should regularly assess their practices and results to identify any inconsistencies or areas for improvement in laboratory operations.
- Furthermore, implementing protocols and training programmes can ensure that all staff members adhere to practices that promote consistency. Regular performance evaluations and feedback also play a role in helping staff members identify areas where they can improve.

Improving success rates is a multi-dimensional issue. Finding a solution may take time and effort to identify and address the underlying reasons for fluctuations. However, by monitoring and improving laboratory practices, ART laboratories can gradually enhance their outcomes over time.

CHAPTER 8

SUMMARY

- Optimal embryo culture conditions are essential for embryo development and survival.
- Monitoring and maintaining the temperature, pH, gas composition, VOCs, culture media, and humidity is necessary.
- Regular quality control checks contribute to successful IVF outcomes by ensuring a stable culture environment.
- Monitoring embryo development helps identify issues and optimises embryo selection for transfer.
- Cleavage-stage embryo evaluation involves assessing cell division, cell size, and fragmentation.
- The evaluation of blastocyst development encompasses observing and analysing the inner cell mass, trophectoderm, and blastocoel cavity.
- Timelapse imaging can provide additional insights into embryo development and aids in selecting high-quality embryos.
- Troubleshooting common embryo culture issues, such as slow or arrested development, fragmentation, and multinucleation, is essential for improving IVF success rates.
- Regular staff training, adherence to established protocols, and thorough documentation can help prevent and resolve issues during embryo culturing.

9

Quality Control in Cryopreservation

9.1 Overview of Cryopreservation

Cryopreservation allows for preserving embryos, oocytes (eggs), and sperm for future use by cooling them to very low temperatures (–196 °C) in liquid nitrogen.

9.2 Procedures

- Storing surplus embryos from IVF for future use.
- Keeping sperm stored in cases where a male partner might have trouble providing a semen sample during egg collection due to medical reasons or personal circumstances.
- Preserving eggs for patients who are about to undergo chemotherapy or radiation therapy that could potentially harm their reproductive organs.
- Protecting testicular tissue for patients who face the risk of infertility due to certain conditions or treatments.

9.3 Fertility Preservation

Fertility preservation involves the storage of eggs, sperm, or embryos for future use. Medical treatments like chemotherapy and radiation therapy can have effects on organs and fertility. In women, these treatments can potentially harm eggs, while men may experience damage to their sperm or testes. Fertility preservation allows individuals to freeze their cells before undergoing treatment, thus improving their likelihood of having children after treatment.

> **Delayed childbearing:** Many people decide to postpone starting a family until later in life. However, it is important to note that a woman's age significantly impacts her fertility, with fertility declining as age increases.

DOI: 10.1201/9781032622736-9

Genetic disorders: Certain genetic conditions, such as Turner syndrome in women and Klinefelter syndrome in men, can make natural conception more challenging due to decreased production of eggs and sperm. In these cases, taking steps for fertility preservation can protect the possibility of having biological children later on.

9.4 Quality Control

Cooling rate: Vitrification uses much higher cooling rates, often exceeding −10,000 °C/min, which aids in maintaining sample viability during cryopreservation.

Storage conditions of frozen sample: Maintain constant storage conditions for cryopreserved gametes, embryos, or tissues at −196 °C. It is advisable to have alarm systems and backup measures in place to mitigate any risks associated with temperature fluctuations.

Warming and viability assessment: The temperature transition from −196 °C to 37 °C occurs at a rapid rate during the warming process of frozen samples. Typically, the warming rate used is approximately 180 °C to 200 °C per minute. After thawing, cell viability can be assessed based on morphological characteristics or other sample-specific practices.

Equipment maintenance: Regular maintenance and calibration of storage tanks and alarm equipment are essential for preserving the quality of stored samples.

Batch consistency: Request certificates from suppliers for every batch, as certificates provide information on quality control testing and batch-specific data. Additionally, cryopreservation media should be stored according to manufacturer recommendations.

Shelf life: Use cryopreservation media within its recommended shelf life. Avoid using expired media to ensure results.

SOPs: Maintain quality standards throughout the cryopreservation and warming process by developing and following SOPs for each stage.

Competency: Prioritise the training and proficiency of embryologists to uphold quality control. Regular assessments, education, and staying updated are crucial for laboratory personnel.

Documentation and tracking: Accurately document all samples, including their identification number, donor or patient information, collection date, processing details, and storage conditions.

Establish a defined sample tracking system that accurately identifies each sample's location and history. This system should include protocols for labelling and tracking samples during handling, processing, and storage as well as document any changes in sample location or status.

QMS: Implementing ISO 9001 or a similar quality management system can help manage and monitor aspects of freezing and warming in ART labs.

9.5 Dilemma of Expired Embryo, Sperm, and Oocyte Storage

The preservation of embryos, sperm, and eggs through freezing has become an important aspect of ART procedures. While the use of cryopreservation techniques has greatly facilitated fertility treatments, it has also presented challenges for fertility clinics worldwide.

Accumulation: The consistent accumulation of cryopreserved embryos, sperm, and oocytes is significant. Following a successful birth, many decide against having more children, leading to the discontinuation of their interest in renewing the storage or donating the embryo to other potential parents or research.

Financial and logistical implications: Maintaining these cryopreserved materials entails not only the cost of storage but also the complexities associated with consistent record-keeping. Clinics bear the burden of storage expenses and also face administrative challenges when managing these records.

The ethical challenge of discarding biological material: Deciding when and how to discard embryos presents an ethical challenge. While many clinics do have a time limit on storage, the act of discarding biological material, especially potential life forms, requires careful consideration.

Patient communication: Reaching out to patients to discuss the future of their stored material is an issue that clinics often encounter. While some individuals play a role in making decisions, others may be more difficult to reach or hesitant to make a choice, resulting in prolonged storage.

Regulatory solutions and informed consent: Regulatory bodies should develop guidelines regarding the duration of storage and the process of obtaining consent for disposal. By updating and clarifying the informed consent procedure, clinics and patients can make informed choices about the future of stored embryos, sperm, and oocytes.

9.6 Troubleshooting Cryopreservation Problems

Thawing efficiency: It is crucial to optimise the thawing process to minimise harm to cells and maintain their viability. During the thawing process, even a small deviation from the recommended thawing rate can impact cell viability. Embryos or oocytes need to be carefully managed during the thawing stage. Cryoprotectants can be harmful at high concentrations, therefore it is important to remove them gradually during the thawing process to prevent any damage to cells.

Ice crystal formation: Ice crystals have the potential to cause damage to the structures and membranes of cells, ultimately leading to their death.

Poor survival rates: If survival rates after thawing are low, it is advisable to evaluate the cryopreservation method in use and consider exploring alternative protocols. Adjusting practices may also help improve outcomes.

Sample mix-ups or losses: To prevent any mix-ups or losses of samples, it is crucial to establish a system for sample identification and tracking that includes labelling and documentation.

Procedural errors: Communication breakdowns among staff members or deviations from established protocols pose risks of losing embryos or gametes in ART laboratories. It is crucial for ART laboratories to establish comprehensive protocols and to ensure that all staff members are trained to adhere to them. Regular reviews are recommended to ensure their accuracy and alignment with advancements in ART fields.

Human error: Common causes of missing embryos or gametes include mislabelling or mishandling. To prevent errors, ART laboratories should implement quality control procedures, including checking labels and documentation, providing staff training, and promoting ongoing education.

Systemic challenges: Missing samples can often be attributed to issues within laboratory settings. Infrastructure, resource limitations, and poor management practices contribute to errors and mismanagement.

To address these issues effectively, laboratories should conduct evaluations of their practices. Basic enhancements must be implemented to create resources and management practices that facilitate sample handling.

Theft, misplacement of samples: It is important to recognise that accidents or errors in cryopreservation can happen, although they are rare. These incidents have the potential to disrupt the aspirations and plans of individuals who depend on preserved samples for their goals. To address this concern, laboratories should implement security measures such as surveillance cameras, access controls, and regular audits. Keycard systems or biometric scanners can restrict entry to certain areas.

9.7 Preventing Embryos or Gametes from Falling under Liquid Nitrogen Storage Tank

Frozen samples falling under the liquid nitrogen tank is a rare occurrence, but it cannot be completely ruled out. This can cause serious problems in cryopreservation.

Improper handling: Improper handling of storage containers is a significant risk factor for the loss of embryos or gametes in ART labs. When canisters are not securely fastened or stored in an environment, they can become unstable and potentially harm the sample. To prevent this problem, ART laboratories should ensure that all storage containers or canisters are securely fastened and kept in a controlled environment. This may involve using racks or shelves designed to support the weight of the containers and securing them with straps or other fasteners to prevent any movement.

Overcrowding: Overcrowding can pose significant challenges in storage facilities. To address this, storage units need to be meticulously constructed and consistently

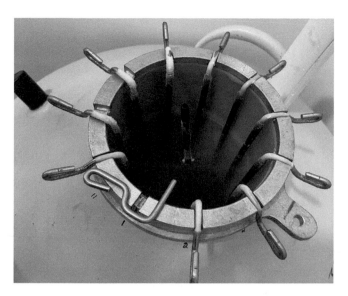

FIGURE 9.1
Photograph showing broken canister.

maintained to bear the load of the items they house, ensuring they don't tilt or collapse. In addition to the structural aspects, there are other critical monitoring tasks to consider.

Equipment failure: A malfunctioning storage tank or a broken canister causes embryos or gametes to fall under liquid nitrogen. To prevent this, ART labs should guarantee that all equipment is properly maintained, calibrated, and regularly inspected for potential issues (Figure 9.1).

Frozen sample management: A lack of guidelines for managing samples can lead to them being misplaced. This uncertainty often forces staff to rely on their judgement, which can lead to mistakes.

It is therefore crucial to establish protocols and procedures to ensure the proper handling of samples. Doing so is not only a duty but also a responsibility towards the individuals and society that these laboratories serve.

9.8 Fear of Reporting Incidents

There is fear among staff about reporting incidents like embryos or gametes accidentally falling into the liquid nitrogen tank. Staff members may be afraid of facing consequences or losing their jobs if they report mishandling or equipment failures. This fear creates a culture of silence where incidents go unreported, putting care and outcomes at risk.

To tackle this problem, it is crucial for ART laboratories to prioritise fostering a culture of transparency and open communication. Staff should feel comfortable reporting incidents without fearing any form of retribution. Laboratory management, embryologists, and clinicians need to establish policies and procedures for incident reporting. Additionally, providing whistleblower protections for staff who come forward with concerns is essential.

9.9 Safety Precautions

Proper ventilation: The laboratory needs to have a well-designed ventilation system that meets its requirements. It is crucial to place the cryostorage tanks in areas that are not confined or have limited airflow.

Oxygen alarm: To ensure safety in the liquid nitrogen storage area, it is crucial to position audible oxygen monitors, particularly near the region where nitrogen gas tends to collect due to its higher density than air. These alarms notify personnel if the oxygen levels drop below a predetermined threshold, typically around 19.5%. In the event of an alarm activation, evacuating the storage area promptly becomes crucial to preventing any risks of asphyxiation.

9.10 Staff Training

- **Operation and maintenance:** It is fundamental that laboratory personnel possess a comprehensive understanding of the manufacturer's guidelines and the ability to diagnose and resolve common issues effectively. Refresher training sessions can be used to reinforce existing knowledge.

9.11 Spill Containment and Cleanup Equipment

- To mitigate damage from LN_2 in the event of a spill, it is recommended to install spill containment barriers or trays beneath the storage containers. Providing absorbent materials is a prerequisite for effectively containing spills.

9.12 Safety Showers

- These stations may help to prevent or minimise the risk of injury to eyes or skin due to accidental exposure to LN_2. Periodic testing of safety showers and eyewash stations is compulsory to ensure their proper functioning and to verify water pressure and temperature adequacy.

9.13 Fire Safety Equipment

- In cryorooms, it is necessary to have fire safety equipment, emergency exits, and evacuation routes in place in ART laboratories where liquid nitrogen is stored and used.
- ART laboratories must guarantee the availability and easy accessibility of fire extinguishers within the lab.

9.14 Emergency Exits and Evacuation Routes

Emergency exits and evacuation routes enable evacuation in case of any emergency situation. It is crucial that these exit routes remain unobstructed and be designed for use. Additionally, all personnel should be familiar with the evacuation procedures.

9.15 Warning Signage

Effective warning signage and reliable emergency alarm systems are components of ART labs that handle nitrogen. These systems play a role in alerting laboratory personnel to hazards. To effectively communicate the message, warning signs should be clear and visible and feature recognised symbols and colours.

9.16 Emergency Response Plan

A comprehensive emergency response plan that defines necessary actions during a crisis ensures personnel safety, secures the lab and equipment, and includes plans for sample relocation if needed is key. Contact information for essential services should be included in the emergency response plan.

9.17 Risk Assessment

Risk assessments should consider potential hazards associated with lab location, infrastructure, and storage equipment, with appropriate safety measures implemented based on identified risks.

Other infrastructure risks should include issues such as power outages, equipment failure, or structural damage that could affect the lab's operation.

Emergency contact list: There should be a comprehensive roster of emergency contacts listing relevant entities such as local authorities, emergency services, and other pertinent organisations.

Safe and secure sample relocation: There should be a transportation plan for relocating cryopreserved samples to suitable alternative storage facilities, ensuring compliance with regulations and guidelines.

9.18 Communication

In case of an emergency, it is essential to have a communication plan in place to coordinate with authorities and emergency services. It is advisable to designate someone within the laboratory as the contact person for all communication efforts.

Ensuring that safety protocols and guidelines are followed is vital to protecting cryopreserved samples and guaranteeing the wellbeing of laboratory staff during emergencies or procedures. Additionally, conducting risk assessments and implementing management strategies play a role in maintaining efficient laboratory operations even in potential disaster situations.

CHAPTER 9

SUMMARY

- Cryopreservation involves preserving embryos, sperm, and oocytes at extremely low temperatures ($-196\ °C$) using liquid nitrogen.
- Quality control is essential to maintaining the viability of preserved gametes and embryos for successful IVF outcomes.
- Proper labelling, storage, and handling of samples are crucial aspects of quality control.
- Cryopreservation in ART has enhanced fertility treatments but introduced challenges to fertility clinics like accumulating stored embryos, financial burdens, logistical complexities, and ethical dilemmas regarding the disposal of potential life forms.
- Performing routine maintenance on cryopreservation equipment is advisable to maintain reliable and consistent performance.
- Resolving problems related to the loss, contamination, or damage of samples during freezing and thawing is paramount.
- Staff training, protocol adherence, and equipment maintenance can minimise cryopreservation problems.
- Preventing embryos or gametes from falling into a liquid nitrogen storage tank involves mitigating human error, equipment failure, and inadequate protocols.
- Implementing secondary containment systems helps to prevent accidents.

- Encouraging a culture of open communication and accountability improves transparency and overall safety in IVF labs.
- It is recommended to periodically review and update protocols to ensure accuracy and alignment with the latest advancements in ART fields.
- Components of an emergency response plan include staff training, clear communication channels, and established protocols for handling various scenarios.

10

Record-Keeping and Documentation

Maintaining detailed records is incredibly important in the healthcare field, as it forms the basis for providing care and service. These records help healthcare professionals keep track of treatment progress, identify areas for improvement, and promptly address any emerging issues. Organised and thorough record-keeping sets the stage for audits, quality assessments, and compliance checks.

Implementing safeguards that protect all records and limit access to authorised personnel is essential. Furthermore, it is vital to have a system in place to report and handle any breaches in data security that may occur while handling sensitive information, like patient records.

10.1 Types of Records

Standardisation: By documenting procedures, protocols, and guidelines, labs can establish an approach that ensures every patient receives the same level of care regardless of who is involved in their treatment. Additionally, proper evaluation yields reproducible results.

Monitoring equipment: Thoroughly documenting equipment maintenance records and usage logs ensures that laboratory equipment works best while preserving the integrity of samples and processes. Accurate equipment documentation also helps to address issues related to equipment performance that could impact both laboratory efficiency and patient outcomes.

To ensure adequate patient care, it is essential to have documented medical and laboratory procedures, protocols, and guidelines. To maintain the functioning of all laboratory equipment, it is important to keep records of equipment calibration, maintenance, and usage logs. Maintaining temperature, humidity, and air quality control and records is crucial for creating appropriate conditions for embryos and gametes.

To ensure the accurate preservation of gametes and embryos for use, documentation of the cryopreservation process, storage conditions, and sample identification is vital. Efficient data management is essential to maintaining well-organised patient records. Therefore, proper documentation related to data management should be maintained. Keeping records that help identify errors or deviations in procedures can significantly contribute to quality control and error reduction. Documentation that allows laboratories to identify bottlenecks and inefficiencies plays a role in optimising laboratory processes. Therefore, workflow records are important.

Effective communication among healthcare professionals involved in ART can be facilitated through documentation that promotes communication. Maintaining precise

DOI: 10.1201/9781032622736-10

financial and administrative records is crucial for managing various facets of the clinic. Proper documentation on the handling and disposal methods for materials reduces the potential for contamination, thereby guaranteeing biosecurity and preventing infections.

Traceability records: These records keep track of where each consumable item and media used in the clinic originates from and its history.

Incident reports: These documents serve as a record of any incidents, near misses, or adverse events that occur, providing information for reference and informing preventive measures.

Legal documents: Consent forms, records of gamete donors, and other relevant documents ensure that the clinic operates within legal guidelines.

Emergency preparedness: The clinic maintains documentation outlining emergency protocols and plans for disaster recovery.

Personnel records: Comprehensive records are kept regarding employee training, certifications, and performance assessments.

Donor screening and selection records: The donor screening process is thoroughly documented to ensure transparency in the selection process.

Research and development records: The testing of techniques and procedures is documented to drive improvements to the clinic's practices.

10.2 Clinical Records

Maintaining records of a patient's history is crucial. This includes information about surgeries, medical conditions, medications, and allergies. These records play a role in assessing treatment options and identifying risks. Obtaining consent, it is essential to document discussions to ensure that patients have an understanding of their treatment choices and can provide consent.

To provide care and closely monitor treatment progress, it is important to document medication protocols and monitoring schedules.

To evaluate treatment effectiveness, recording ultrasound monitoring results such as growth measurements, endometrial thickness, and follicular count is vital. These records also serve as information for making any adjustments to the treatment plan. Proper documentation of medication management is essential for therapy. This includes documenting dosage instructions, timing of administration, and potential side effects. Such documentation plays a role in evaluating treatment outcomes.

Additionally, it is crucial to document any events experienced by patients during ART procedures. Paying attention to allergic reactions, incidents, or infections helps ensure safety while providing necessary information for future treatments. Collecting and documenting patient feedback is crucial for ART labs to identify areas where they can improve patient care services; this in turn enhances their experience by effectively addressing their specific needs. During follow-up care, it is important to keep records of pregnancy and delivery outcomes. This helps in evaluating the long-term success of ART procedures and providing support for patients.

Having documentation of genetic counselling sessions is essential. These sessions cover topics such as risks, benefits, informed consent, and proper selection of testing. In this way, patients are fully aware of how these tests may impact future generations.

To prepare for clinic closures, a plan outlining the steps is needed. This includes arrangements for transferring patients to alternative clinics and ensuring the storage and disposal of specimens and records.

Implementing policies regarding document retention is essential and helps maintain order by specifying how long records should be retained and where they should be stored and ensuring compliance with laws and regulations.

10.3 Document Control

Effective document control is part of correct management of documents. It involves handling stages like creation, review, approval, distribution, and preservation to gather information and safeguard sensitive data. Another significant aspect of data management is archiving and retrieval. This involves organising and accessing physical documents in a manner to ensure easy retrieval when needed.

Maintaining document control plays a role in laboratory management and requires the establishment of policies and procedures that are regularly reviewed to keep them up to date and effective. Electronic document management systems are often utilised for this purpose. These systems act as a centralised repository for all documentation, making it easier to access, monitor, and make modifications as needed and thereby improving efficiency and control.

10.4 Standard Operating Procedures

10.4.1 Development and Implementation

10.4.1.1 Process Mapping

Process mapping involves outlining all the steps and activities carried out in the laboratory, including collecting and processing samples, conducting analyses, and performing procedures. Creating a detailed process map that covers all aspects of patient care is a task that forms the foundation for operations and excellent services for patients.

Risk assessment: Risks can be identified using methods such as flowcharts, fault trees, or failure mode and effects analyses (see Chapter 3).

Risk ranking: Giving priority to risks with high impact ensures that they receive proper attention and mitigation measures are put in place.

10.5 Define the Scope and Purpose of Each SOP

It ensures that all relevant aspects of a process or procedure are thoroughly covered. This clarity also guarantees that the SOP provides concise guidance to laboratory personnel, promoting consistency and reliability for achieving the desired outcomes.

10.6 Process of Defining Scope and Purpose

Identify the specific process: This should be accomplished through rigorous process mapping and risk assessment.

Determine the intended outcomes: The intended outcomes of the process or procedure should be clearly defined. It comprises improving patient outcomes, increasing lab efficiency, reducing errors or variability, and complying with regulatory requirements.

Develop a consistent format and structure: Creating a consistent format and structure for the SOPs in an ART laboratory can streamline the process, making it easier for staff to understand and adhere to protocols.

A typical SOP might include the following.

Title: The title should be descriptive and accurately reflect the process or procedure being covered in the SOP.

Objective: An explanation for the procedure, ensuring that everyone involved understands why the measure is being taken and what results are expected. A clear statement helps to align all stakeholders and personnel, ensuring that everyone recognises the importance of the procedure and the desired outcomes.

Responsibilities: Precise information on who is responsible for each stage of the procedure, including quality control.

Procedure: A detailed, step-by-step description of the process of safety precautions, equipment settings, or quality control measures. This section should provide clear and concise instructions for specific requirements or details critical to success.

Reference documents: A list of relevant guidelines, standards, or regulations based on the SOP. This section should recognise any external sources of information or guidance used in developing the SOP.

Definitions: A glossary of any specialised terms or abbreviations used in the SOP. This section should provide definitions for any terms or abbreviations that may be unfamiliar or confusing to staff.

Revision history: A record of all modifications to the SOP, comprising the date, a summary of the alteration, and the individual accountable for the revision. This section aims to facilitate staff awareness of any modifications made to the SOP and provide access to previous versions if needed.

10.7 Use Clear and Concise Language

Effective communication is vital when it comes to writing SOPs. It is important to avoid using jargon or complex language, as this can lead to confusion and errors. By keeping the language clear and straightforward, SOPs become easier to write and quicker to read, ultimately enhancing efficiency and compliance.

10.8 Visual Aids and Examples

To enhance understanding and identify any errors or inefficiencies, visual aids like flowcharts, diagrams, and photographs can be incredibly helpful. Additionally, providing examples of completed forms or records can ensure documentation.

> **Completed forms or records:** This contains examples of patient information forms, laboratory reports, or quality control records. Staff members can use these examples as a reference when completing their forms or records, ensuring that all necessary information is included.

10.9 Establish a Document Control System

A document control system maintains the integrity and accuracy of SOPs.

This system should assign identifiers to each version while ensuring that only the most up-to-date version is in use. Removing versions is crucial to preventing confusion and errors.

10.10 Train Staff on SOPs and Assess Competency

Training employees plays a role in ensuring that they understand and adhere to SOPs. It is important to assess their competency after training through tests or practical demonstrations to confirm their ability to carry out procedures accurately.

10.11 Monitor Compliance and Performance

Regularly monitoring compliance and performance through audits, observation, and tracking performance indicators helps evaluate the effectiveness of procedures while identifying areas for improvement.

10.12 Continuously Review and Update SOPs

SOPs must undergo reviews and updates based on scheduled reviews, changes in regulations, technological advancements, or best practices. During this process, it is crucial to consider input from staff regarding the practicality and effectiveness of SOPs.

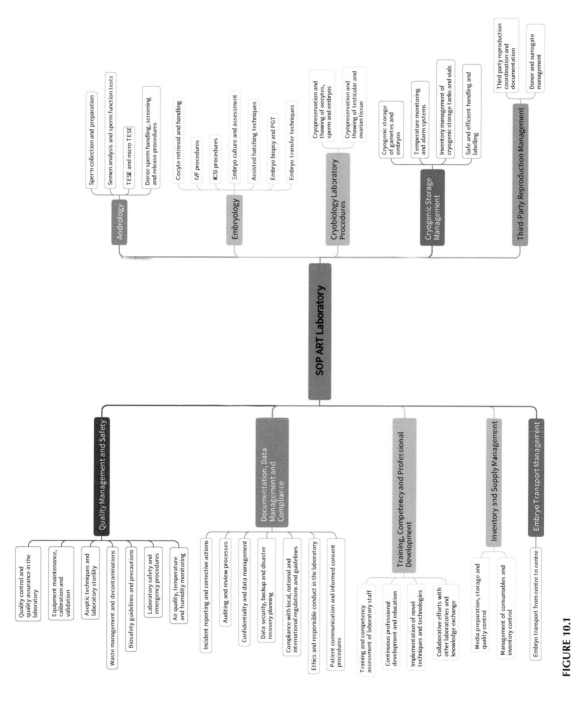

FIGURE 10.1
Flowchart showing an overview of the SOP list.

10.13 Comprehensive ART Laboratory SOP List

Every ART laboratory needs comprehensive SOPs to ensure procedural success. This includes practices in andrology, embryology, and cryobiology, with a focus on tasks from sperm collection to embryo transfer. Proper cryogenic storage management, third-party reproduction coordination, and rigorous quality and safety protocols are essential. Data management ensures secure and ethical communication, while continuous staff training and efficient inventory management optimise operations. Moreover, safe embryo transport between centres is paramount. Specific protocols may vary depending on the laboratory, equipment, and individual case requirements.

10.14 Sample Standard Operating Procedure for an ART Lab Procedure

Note that this is just an example of an SOP, and the specific steps, equipment, and parameters may vary depending on the lab and the density gradient medium used. Always consult the manufacturer's instructions for the specific products used in the lab and follow the lab's guidelines and accreditation requirements.

SAMPLE 1: SPERM PREPARATION: DENSITY GRADIENT

Title: Sperm Preparation—Double-Layer Density Gradient Centrifugation

Objective: To isolate motile, morphologically normal sperm from raw semen samples for use in assisted reproductive procedures.

Scope: This SOP applies to all laboratory personnel involved in sperm preparation following the density gradient centrifugation method.

Responsibilities: Embryologists and andrology technicians are responsible for performing the procedure according to this SOP; the laboratory supervisor is responsible for ensuring compliance with the SOP and addressing any issues that arise.

Procedure

- Centrifuge
- Sterile conical tubes (15 mL)
- Sterile pipettes
- Density gradient medium (e.g., 40% and 80% solutions)
- Sperm wash media

Preparation of Culture Media

- Pre-warm the culture media to 37 °C in a water bath or incubator.
- Label a sterile 15 mL conical tube with the patient's identification and unique number.

- Gently mix the raw semen sample.
- In a sterile 15 mL conical tube, carefully layer 1 mL of the 80% density gradient medium.
- Gently layer 1 mL of the 40% density gradient medium on top of the 80% layer, creating a two-layer gradient.
- Carefully layer 1 mL of the liquefied semen sample on top of the 40% density gradient medium layer.
- Centrifuge the conical tube at 2,000 RPM for 20 minutes at room temperature.
- After centrifugation, carefully remove the supernatant and the two layers of density gradient medium, leaving the pellet of sperm at the bottom of the tube.
- Add 2 mL of sperm washing medium to the conical tube and gently resuspend the sperm pellet.
- Centrifuge the conical tube at room temperature again at 300× g for 10 minutes.
- Remove the supernatant, leaving the final sperm pellet.
- Resuspend the final sperm pellet in an appropriate volume of sperm washing medium or culture medium, depending on the intended use.
- Assess the pre- and post-preparation sperm sample for concentration, motility, and morphology and document the results.

Reference documents: *WHO Laboratory Manual for the Examination and Processing of Human Semen*, 2010.

Definitions

- **RPM**: Rotations per minute, or the force exerted on a sample during centrifugation, expressed as a multiple of the Earth's gravitational force (g).
- **Supernatant**: The liquid remaining after a solid has settled during centrifugation.

Revision History

- Version 1.0: [Date]—Initial development and approval.
- Version 1.1: [Date]—Updated centrifugation parameters based on new equipment.

SAMPLE 2: SPERM PREPARATION: SWIM-UP TECHNIQUE

Objective: To isolate motile sperm from a semen sample sperm for use in IUI and IVF/ICSI.

Scope: This SOP applies to all laboratory personnel performing sperm preparation using the swim-up technique in the ART lab.

Responsibilities: Personnel in the laboratory are accountable for carrying out the procedure, keeping accurate records, and ensuring compliance with this SOP. The laboratory supervisor supervises the technique and ensures all personnel are adequately trained and competent in its execution.

Procedure

Semen sample collection and liquefaction: instruct the patient to obtain the semen in a sterile container. Allow the sample to liquefy for 20 to 30 minutes at ambient temperature.

Preparation of Culture Media

- Pre-warm the culture media to 37 °C in a water bath or incubator.
- Label a sterile 15 mL conical tube with the patient's identification.

Swim-Up Technique

- Carefully transfer 1 mL of the liquefied semen sample to the bottom of the conical tube using a micropipette.
- Slowly layer 1 mL of pre-warmed culture media on top of the semen sample; avoid mixing the layers.
- Incubate the conical tube at an angle of approximately 45° for 60 minutes at 37 °C.
- After incubation, carefully aspirate the top 0.8 mL of culture media containing the motile sperm using a micropipette.
- Transfer the aspirated media, which contains the motile sperm, to a sterile tube labelled with the patient's identification.

Sperm Concentration and Motility Assessment

- Assess the sperm concentration and motility of the pre- and post-preparation sample using a Maklar chamber and a phase-contrast microscope.
- Record the results in the appropriate laboratory form.

Reference Documents

- World Health Organisation. (2010). *WHO Laboratory Manual for the Examination and Processing of Human Semen* (5th ed.). World Health Organisation.
- [Any additional guidelines, standards, or regulatory documents relevant to your lab].
- Definitions:
    1. IUI: Intrauterine insemination
    2. IVF: In vitro fertilisation

Revision History

- Version 1.0: [Date]—Initial version of SOP.
- [Any subsequent changes (the date, description of the change and the person responsible for the update.)]
- Please note that this model SOP is for illustrative purposes only and should be adapted to fit the specific needs, regulations, and guidelines applicable to the ART lab.

SAMPLE 3: INTRACYTOPLASMIC SPERM INJECTION (ICSI)

Purpose: To provide a standard operating procedure for ICSI in the embryology laboratory to ensure this assisted reproductive technique's consistency, quality, and safety.

Scope: This SOP applies to all embryology laboratory staff performing ICSI.

Responsibilities: Embryology laboratory staff are responsible for following this SOP and ensuring that proper aseptic technique is maintained during all procedures.

Materials and Equipment

- Sterile work area (laminar flow hood)
- Inverted microscope with micromanipulators
- Sterile culture dishes, 4.4 micropipettes and tips
- Holding and injection pipettes
- Incubator
- Oocyte collection and sperm preparation materials
- Sterile culture media

Procedure

Oocyte and sperm preparation:

Collect mature oocytes by standard oocyte retrieval methods.

Prepare sperm samples using appropriate sperm preparation techniques (e.g., swim-up or density gradient centrifugation).

Denuding Oocytes

- Prepare a sterile dish with hyaluronidase enzyme solution.

Transfer the oocytes to the enzyme solution and incubate for a short time (approximately 30–60 seconds) to remove the surrounding cumulus cells.

- Transfer the denuded oocytes to a dish containing culture media and assess for maturity.

Performing ICSI

- Transfer mature oocytes to an ICSI dish containing droplets of sperm, polyvinylpyrrolidone (PVP) solution, and culture media.
- Select a single, motile sperm and immobilise it by breaking its tail through the injection pipette.
- Hold the oocyte in place using the holding pipette and insert the injection pipette through the zona pellucida and lemma.
- Inject the sperm into the oocyte cytoplasm and carefully withdraw the injection pipette.

Post-ICSI Culture and Assessment

- Transfer the injected oocytes to a culture dish and incubate under controlled temperature, humidity, and CO_2 levels.
- Assess the oocytes for fertilisation approximately 16–20 hours after ICSI.
- Monitor the development of fertilised oocytes daily and grade embryos based on established criteria.

Quality Control and Documentation

- Maintain detailed records of all ICSI procedures, including oocyte and sperm preparation, injection parameters, and fertilisation outcomes.
- Review and update the SOP periodically based on new information, techniques, and technologies.

Safety Precautions

- Handle oocytes and sperm with care and follow appropriate biosafety guidelines.
- Wear appropriate personal protective equipment (gloves, lab coat, and safety goggles).
- Dispose of all waste materials according to laboratory guidelines and regulations.

References: Relevant references and guidelines for ICSI, laboratory procedures, and safety protocols.

Revision History

- Version 1.0: [Date]—Initial development and approval.
- Version 1.1: [Date]—Updated centrifugation parameters based on new equipment.

CHAPTER 10

SUMMARY

- Accurate record-keeping and documentation are essential for quality, safety, and traceability in ART clinics.
- Records and documents include patient records, informed consent forms, laboratory data, equipment maintenance logs, and quality control records.
- Proper document control ensures the use of up-to-date and approved documents.
- Archiving records and documents allow for easy retrieval and review, which is crucial for audits and legal purposes.
- An organised system should be in place for storing, managing, and retrieving records and documents.
- SOPs are detailed instructions for performing specific tasks consistently and safely in ART labs.
- SOPs help maintain quality, reduce errors, and guarantee compliance with regulations and guidelines.
- Developing SOPs includes identifying procedures, gathering input from staff, and writing clear instructions.
- Implementing SOPs requires staff training, monitoring adherence, and regular review and updates.
- Sample SOPs for ART lab procedures should contain the purpose, materials, equipment, step-by-step instructions, and precautions.

11

QC of ART Labs Personnel

The effectiveness of an ART laboratory heavily relies on the skills and expertise of its personnel. Staff have responsibilities such as managing gametes and embryos and operating laboratory equipment. To stay up to date with advancements in science and reproductive medicine, it is vital for the lab team to engage in learning through seminars, webinars, and workshops. Gaining certifications from organisations like the American Board of Bioanalysis, American Association of Bioanalysts, ESHERE, IFS, and ISAR also adds to their credibility. Regular monitoring of their performance involves observing their work, reviewing records and documentation, and tracking key performance indicators. It is crucial to assess their proficiency in evaluating embryo quality and interpreting results. Having SOPs for every process within the IVF lab is essential. Adhering to SOPs contributes to evaluating their performance. Since dealing with IVF also involves considerations such as informed consent, patient confidentiality, and proper handling of embryos, training should also cover these aspects.

11.1 Importance of Personnel QC in ART Labs

The skills mentioned have an impact on patients' well-being. It is also crucial for staff members to be prepared for situations like power outages or equipment failures that could potentially put the safety of embryos at risk.

Trained staff who can perform laboratory procedures accurately and precisely play a role in ensuring accuracy and precision. Regular training and evaluation ensure that staff members adhere to established processes and deliver results.

Consistency is key in achieving long-term success in ART laboratories, as even minor variations can affect outcomes. Staff members follow protocols that consistently lead to dependable results.

Compliance with guidelines is essential for ART laboratories. Although human error may occasionally occur, personnel quality control measures minimise mistakes by ensuring that staff members receive training and strictly follow protocols (Figure 11.1).

11.2 Personnel Training and Qualifications

It is vital to have a trained and qualified team in an ART lab to ensure accuracy and consistency. When professionals in these labs possess an understanding of their craft, they effectively carry out the procedures that are crucial for the success of ART; this is why continuous learning and qualifications have a role in this field.

DOI: 10.1201/9781032620726-11

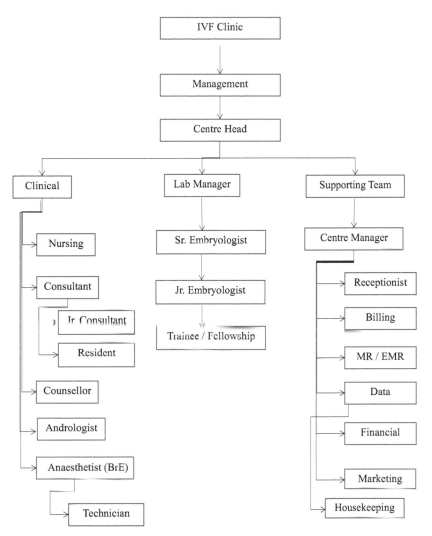

FIGURE 11.1
Overview of standard team members in a fertility clinic.

ART lab director: The position of a laboratory director is crucial, as they oversee all operations within the laboratory. One important aspect of their role is ensuring that personnel receive training and earn qualifications, which the director must continuously monitor. To effectively carry out these responsibilities, it is ideal for the laboratory director to have a postgraduate degree in the sciences or life sciences. Alternatively, a degree in management sciences could equip them with the leadership skills and organisational knowledge necessary for managing the lab.

Infertility specialist: It is essential for ART specialists to hold a postgraduate degree in gynaecology and obstetrics, as this provides them with the knowledge necessary for their role. Additionally, clinicians must undergo training in ART procedures through recognised programmes that lead to certification.

Embryologists: Embryologists perform tasks such as semen analysis, sperm preparation, oocyte screening, IVF, ICSI, embryo culture, embryo transfer, embryo biopsy, and cryobiology. To excel in this multifaceted role, embryologists need a postgraduate degree in embryology, or a postgraduate degree in the life sciences combined with training can also suffice.

Embryologists require about four years of experience to effectively apply their theoretical knowledge in real-life scenarios. Specialised training programmes focusing on ART procedures ensure that embryologists are well versed in the techniques and protocols followed in the ART lab.

Andrologists are professionals who specialise in male infertility and surgical sperm retrieval procedures. They hold degrees in MCh or DNB and have received additional training to perform surgical techniques such as TESA, PESA, and TESE.

Technologists have the task of maintaining equipment and supplies within ART laboratories while also conducting routine semen analysis and preparation procedures. Typically, they hold a bachelor's degree in life sciences. They have undergone training through recognised programmes that focus on ART laboratory procedures.

Nurses: To work as nurses in an ART clinic, individuals must possess a diploma or graduate degree, have local nursing council registration, and receive training in ART procedures from accredited programmes.

Psychological counsellors: Counsellors offer support and guidance to patients as they navigate through fertility treatments. The psychologist's role goes beyond giving information; they act as companions during the emotional struggles that often come during fertility journeys. By coordinating with the medical team, they can offer support in handling stress, anxiety, and depression. They explain the various options available and empower patients to make informed choices about their fertility treatment. To pursue a career as a counsellor in this field, having a bachelor's degree is crucial. This degree can be in psychology, which allows for understanding emotions and behaviours, or in fields like social work or nursing to develop caregiving skills.

Housekeeping staff: These dedicated individuals are responsible for maintaining cleanliness and disinfecting all surfaces within the clinic, including floors, walls, counters, and equipment. Their efforts create a safe environment for both staff members and patients and uphold waste management practices. They also play a role in providing guidance to laboratory staff regarding cleaning techniques and safety protocols specific to their work environment. Through training programmes, they become proficient in maintaining suitable laboratory conditions.

11.3 Competency Assessment

The competency of staff members working in ART labs is regularly assessed to ensure they possess the skills, knowledge, and capabilities required for their roles.

This assessment helps identify both areas of strength and areas that need improvement, allowing for training and development opportunities. Job analysis is conducted to gain an understanding of the tasks, responsibilities, equipment, and procedures associated with each position within ART labs. This analysis ensures that clear expectations are set and provides benchmarks for evaluating the competencies of staff members. Training and education programmes are customised to address the needs of staff members working in ART labs. These programmes focus on adhering to regulations and standards set by organisations such as CAP, ASRM, CLIA, and ESHRE.

In India, organisations that oversee the training and education of personnel employed in ART laboratories include the Indian Council of Medical Research (ICMR), the National Accreditation Board for Hospitals and Healthcare Providers, the Federation of Obstetric and Gynaecological Societies of India (FOGSI), the Indian Society for Assisted Reproduction, and the National Board (NA).

11.4 Evaluation

It is essential to keep a record of competency assessments in the personnel files. This record should include the assessment date, the obtained results, and any areas for improvement. Creating a workplace culture that encourages employee feedback and active participation in training and education is crucial to maintaining staff's expertise.

11.5 Job Descriptions and Responsibilities

To ensure clarity and minimise confusion while aligning everyone with common goals, job descriptions play a key role. They provide staff members with an understanding of their roles, responsibilities, and expectations. Job descriptions help streamline work by defining tasks and allowing staff members to focus on their areas of expertise; this promotes coordination among team members and ultimately leads to better efficiency. By working towards shared objectives, the ART lab can achieve desired outcomes efficiently and within given timelines.

Moreover, job descriptions are crucial in setting the expectations for each position. They ensure that individuals are properly trained and have the skills to carry out their assigned tasks successfully.

Fostering growth opportunities: Growth opportunities play a role in facilitating career development by identifying areas for improvement and offering a path for advancement. They serve as a tool for nurturing skills and supporting career progression within the organisation.

11.6 Development of Personnel QC Programme

The personnel QC programme guarantees that staff members possess the skills, reliability, and accuracy required for performing lab procedures. By emphasising precision and consistency through the QC programme, standards of quality and reliability are maintained.

Goals and objectives: To establish a personnel QC programme, the first step is to define its objectives. These goals should be specific, measurable, achievable, relevant, and time-bound (SMART).

Scope: Scope involves identifying the covered laboratory procedures and clearly outlining staff roles and responsibilities. It also entails deciding which types of QC tests will be utilised. To ensure success, it is crucial to develop a training plan that covers aspects such as laboratory procedures, aseptic techniques, and regulatory requirements.

Training plan: The training plan comprises competency assessments, proficiency testing exercises, internal quality control measures, environmental monitoring efforts, and ongoing education for staff members.

Monitoring: Evaluating the personnel QC programme is essential to ensuring that it effectively achieves its goals. This consists of tracking staff competence levels, error rates in procedures performed by them, satisfaction levels with their services, and compliance with established standards.

11.7 Performance Evaluations

To support the growth and development of staff members, various assessments, such as self-assessments, peer evaluations, and performance-based assessments, are conducted. It is also crucial for ART lab staff to stay up to date on advancements in reproductive medicine techniques and procedures through continuing education. This can be achieved by participating in conferences, workshops, online courses, and webinars and by reading literature and research studies. By seeking opportunities for learning and growth, ART laboratory staff can continuously enhance their knowledge and expertise to provide patient care.

11.8 Training Nascent Embryologists

Training budding embryologists is crucial because it provides insight into the various stages of life. Becoming an embryologist requires training that combines learning with valuable hands-on experience over a span of years. This comprehensive training aims to cultivate an understanding of life creation processes while nurturing skills like attention to detail, patience, and ethical awareness.

Embryologists occupy a position at the intersection of science and the creation of life, giving them the ability to shape this journey. Considering their role, their training process is thorough and multifaceted. Continuous professional development and staying up to date with advancements are central aspects of an embryologist's career.

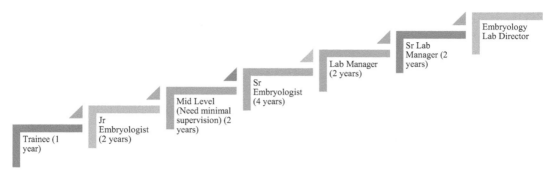

FIGURE 11.2
Professional development in clinical embryology.

11.9 Professional Development in Clinical Embryology

In the field of embryology, career progression begins with a one-year trainee position, where individuals learn the principles and techniques of embryology under supervision. Afterward, they can progress to the role of junior embryologist over the next two years. This phase is marked by developing competence in procedures and taking on new responsibilities

The following two-year period as a mid-level embryologist involves handling a range of procedures, often with minimal supervision. With four years of experience, embryologists can become senior embryologists. In this role, they demonstrate high-level expertise, supervise staff members, and contribute to quality control initiatives in the lab.

After another two years, there is an opportunity for advancement to lab manager. As lab managers, individuals are responsible for overseeing lab operations, ensuring compliance with regulations, and managing both staff and budgets. In this position, they oversee labs or larger facilities while contributing to planning within their institution.

At the pinnacle of their career path lies the role of embryology lab director. Individuals in this position bear responsibility for all aspects of lab operations, including adherence to regulations and ethical guidelines. They also steer research directives within the lab.

It is important to note that this career path assumes that one works consistently in a laboratory setting. However, there are also career options such as research, academia, or policy development. Each of these paths has its own timeline and requirements for advancement.

In the field of embryology, career progression requires more than just experience; one also needs to develop competencies, leadership skills, and management skills for higher-level roles. The timelines provided here are estimates and can vary depending on performance, professional development opportunities, and the job market situation (Figure 11.2).

11.10 Role of Senior Embryologists/Lab Managers in Training

Embryologists and laboratory managers are instrumental in training individuals in ART laboratories. They act as mentors, sharing their knowledge and experience to help trainees develop professionally. Their responsibilities extend beyond teaching to provide

TABLE 11.1

Sample 1: ART Lab Training Logbook – Weekly

Name: Mr John
Level of training: Primary
Supervisor: Mr Smith

Procedure	No. of cases observed	No. of cases done with supervision	No. of cases done independently	Match with senior/ colleagues	Corrective actions	Comments senior	OK to proceed Yes/No
SA	50	40	25	23	nil	ok	Yes
Egg collection	10	1	1	1	More practice	Need more supervision	No
IVF	3	–	–	–	–	–	–

guidance during real-time operations, ensuring that trainees gain an understanding of quality control measures. This encompasses aspects of laboratory operations, including the handling of gametes and embryos and the meticulous maintenance and calibration of equipment.

Training also emphasises the importance of documentation procedures and the ability to analyse records. With oversight and detailed feedback, experienced professionals ensure that trainees can accurately monitor their performance and make improvements. This rigorous approach serves to enhance skills while nurturing an environment that prioritises continuous learning and growth (Table 11.1).

11.11 Skills and Qualities Required for an Embryologist

Being an embryologist is a commitment; it requires a combination of expertise, cognitive abilities, and emotional intelligence. The job demands precision and attention to detail, since minor oversights can have implications for embryo viability and the effectiveness of fertility treatments. It also requires patience due to time-consuming procedures that necessitate high levels of concentration and focus.

Staying updated with research and technological advancements is important for an embryologist. They achieve this by attending conferences, subscribing to journals, and actively participating in networks.

Given the nature of their work, having an ethical compass is crucial for embryologists. They often encounter challenging decisions regarding embryo handling, genetic testing implications, and patient confidentiality. It is important for them to show empathy towards patients who are going through stress due to fertility struggles.

Collaboration and teamwork skills are essential in an ART lab. Embryologists need to coordinate with professionals such as andrologists, reproductive endocrinologists, geneticists, nurses, and lab technicians. They should be capable of explaining procedures to patients and skilled in conflict resolution and problem-solving.

Effective time management skills, decision-making abilities, technological proficiency, resilience, and research skills are also vital for embryologists' professional success. These attributes play a role in keeping up with developments in this field.

11.12 Staff Well-Being and Lab Performance

The well-being of staff members directly impacts the quality of service and productivity in an ART lab. Rested and less stressed workers generally tend to be more effective, precise, and attentive, resulting in enhanced outcomes for ART procedures.

In a field that highly values expertise, it is crucial to maintain a work environment that places importance on employees' well-being. This aids in retaining individuals, reduces turnover rates, and ensures smooth continuity of care, thus directly impacting the success of the laboratory.

11.13 Impact of Stress

Persistent stress can significantly influence an individual's performance in an ART laboratory, harming their ability to concentrate, make decisions, and carry out tasks accurately. Given the nature of ART procedures, even a momentary lapse in focus can have consequences. Chronic stress can result in burnout, characterised by exhaustion, a diminished sense of accomplishment, and a loss of identity. Stress often leads to increased absenteeism and high staff turnover rates, disrupting lab operations and diminishing its success rate.

To address this issue effectively, it is vital to cultivate an environment that prioritises employee comfort and productivity; this includes designing workspaces with appropriate lighting to reduce eye strain as well as fostering a culture that promotes teamwork, mutual respect, and open communication.

11.14 Evaluating a Welfare Programme

Implementing a welfare programme within the ART lab can be an effective approach to promoting employee well-being. It involves conducting check-ins with the team's training managers to recognise signs of stress or burnout among colleagues and offering resources like counselling or stress management workshops.

To ensure the effectiveness of these initiatives, it is crucial to gather feedback from staff members, closely monitor absenteeism and staff turnover rates, and observe any changes in the lab's performance metrics. Prioritising strategies for supporting staff well-being and managing stress is a strategic imperative for delivering top-notch ART services.

CHAPTER 11

SUMMARY

- Implementation of personnel quality control is of paramount importance for maintaining quality and safety in ART laboratories.

- Staff proficiency and consistency in ART procedures are ensured by comprehensive competency assessments.

- Clear job descriptions and responsibilities enhance efficiency by helping staff understand their roles.

- A QC programme includes job descriptions, training, qualification requirements, competency assessments, and performance evaluations, with regular updates necessary for compliance with current guidelines and best practices.

- Continuing education requirements ensure that staff remain current with the latest advances in ART.

- Clear communication and teamwork are vital for efficient workflow and error reduction.

- A mentorship or buddy system supports new staff members and facilitates knowledge transfer.

- Staff meetings provide a platform for discussing issues, sharing updates, and fostering a positive work environment.

- Encouraging staff participation in professional associations and conferences can expand their knowledge and professional network.

- A system for reporting and learning from errors or near misses can improve lab safety and performance.

- Promoting a culture of continuous improvement can enhance the lab's overall quality.

- The role of an embryologist blends theoretical knowledge, practical skills, and essential habits like meticulousness, patience, continuous learning, and teamwork.

- Senior embryologists play a crucial role in training juniors in practical tasks and quality control principles, shaping professionals who uphold high standards in ART.

- Staff well-being and effective stress management strategies are essential for high-quality service delivery, productivity, and strong success rates in ART labs.

12

Key Performance Indicators

KPIs serve as reference points in fertility clinics, helping experts assess the effectiveness of treatments in reaching desired goals, such as pregnancies or live births. To gather KPI data, fertility clinics may perform interviews, review records, and conduct laboratory tests. These data points are thoroughly evaluated to determine how well treatment strategies and interventions are working.

The Vienna consensus contributes to standardising practices in fertility clinics by defining KPIs, recommending data collection methodologies, and underscoring the importance of adjusting data based on variables such as patient age and medical history. The consensus also highlights reporting methods and adjustments, resulting in comprehensive and fair performance assessments across clinics.

Quality control is another aspect that requires fertility clinic teams to understand the significance of KPIs in achieving their goals. Regular supervision of data collection processes can help and involve spot-checking data entries, validating sources for accuracy, and ensuring adherence to established protocols.

Equally crucial is reviewing and assessing the procedures, calculations, and statistical analyses involved in data analysis to consider any factors that may impact results. Ensuring that staff receive training and certification is vital for maintaining the reliability of data collection and analysis. Additionally, fostering an environment that promotes communication and feedback can help identify areas where processes can be improved. By refining these processes based on the feedback received, the overall quality of the data can be consistently improved over time.

12.1 Leveraging Technology for KPI Tracking and Analysis

Electronic health records (EHRs) have an impact in the industry, as they offer a centralised and standardised system for documenting, storing, and conveniently retrieving essential patient data, which makes it easier for fertility specialists to analyse KPIs. When combined with data analytics software, these digital records can be automatically analysed to identify trends, gain insights, and account for any factors that may affect results. Additionally, incorporating telemedicine and remote monitoring technologies allows for real-time tracking of progress and treatment outcomes. Last, implementing data formats and interoperable systems promotes data exchange between different healthcare providers and software platforms.

DOI: 10.1201/9781032622736-12

12.2 Vienna Consensus Guidelines

The Vienna consensus, established in 2017 by a panel of fertility experts, serves as a framework for documenting and evaluating fertility outcomes. Its primary aim is to enhance transparency and precision in fertility research and practice. The formulation of these guidelines involved the collaboration of more than 40 specialists hailing from 28 countries.

This framework ensures that centres are consistently improving outcomes and maintaining standards of care. The guidelines also support the use of KPIs for benchmarking and continuous improvement, allowing clinics and laboratories to compare their performance against established standards, identify areas for enhancement, and track progress over time.

12.3 Development of KPIs

Developing KPIs for assessing and managing infertility is crucial in the field of ART. KPIs provide metrics for embryologists to evaluate the effectiveness of treatment methods (Table 12.1).

12.4 Clinical KPIs

In clinical KPIs, one important metric to consider is the number of eggs retrieved per patient or cumulatively across cycles. This metric provides insight into the efficiency of the egg retrieval process. Another crucial success indicator is clinical pregnancy rate (CPR), or the ratio of pregnancies to the number of embryo transfer procedures. Live birth rate (LBR) represents the proportion of births resulting from ART cycles and is a measure of overall treatment success. Implantation rate (IR) is a measure that reveals the proportion of transferred embryos and provides information about the quality of the embryos and the effectiveness of the transfer technique. Miscarriage rate (MR) indicates the proportion of pregnancies that result in miscarriage. These rates give insights into both the safety and effectiveness of treatments. Considering these metrics together provides an evaluation of a fertility clinic's performance.

12.5 Laboratory KPIs

One important measure in the ART lab is the oocyte maturity rate (OMR), which allows direct assessment of the quality of oocytes during ICSI and aids in evaluating the success of stimulation protocols.

Methods used in sperm preparation, such as density gradient centrifugation and swim-up techniques, influence the quality of sperm samples. Fertilisation rate (FR) is a metric

TABLE 12.1

List of KPIs and Formulas in ART Labs

KPI	Formula	Description
Clinical pregnancy rate (CPR)	(Number of clinical pregnancies/ number of embryo transfers) × 100	Measures the percentage of embryo transfers that result in a clinical pregnancy
Live birth rate (LBR)	(Number of live births/number of embryo transfers) × 100	Calculates the percentage of embryo transfers that result in a live birth
Implantation rate (IR)	(Number of gestational sacs observed/number of embryos transferred) × 100	Measures the percentage of embryos transferred that successfully implant in the uterus and form a gestational sac
Cycle cancellation rate (CCR)	(Number of cancelled cycles/total number of initiated cycles) × 100	Evaluates the percentage of initiated ART cycles that are cancelled before embryo transfer, typically due to poor response, no fertilisation, or other complications
Multiple pregnancy rate (MPR)	(Number of multiple pregnancies/ number of clinical pregnancies) × 100	Measures the percentage of clinical pregnancies that result in multiple gestations (e.g., twins, triplets)
Cumulative live birth rate (CLBR)	(Cumulative number of live births/ number of patients initiating treatment) × 100	Evaluates the overall success of an ART lab by measuring the percentage of patients who achieve a live birth after a complete treatment cycle, including all fresh and frozen embryo transfers
ICSI damage rate	(Number of damaged oocytes/total number of oocytes injected) × 100	Measures the percentage of oocytes that are damaged during the ICSI procedure
IVF normal fertilisation rate	(Number of normally fertilised oocytes/total number of oocytes inseminated) × 100	Assesses the percentage of oocytes that are fertilised normally following conventional IVF
Fertilisation rate (FR)	(Number of fertilised oocytes/ number of oocytes retrieved) × 100	Measures the percentage of oocytes successfully fertilised in an ART cycle
Failed fertilisation rate (IVF)	(Number of failed fertilisation/total number of oocytes inseminated) × 100	Measures the percentage of oocytes that fail to fertilise following IVF
Cleavage rate	(Number of embryos with two or more cells on day 2/total number of fertilised oocytes) × 100	Measures the percentage of fertilised oocytes that develop into embryos with two or more cells on day 2
Blastocyst formation rate	(Number of blastocysts formed/total number of fertilised oocytes) × 100	Measures the percentage of fertilised oocytes that develop into blastocysts
Successful biopsy rate	(Number of successful biopsies/total number of attempted biopsies) × 100	Evaluates the percentage of biopsies that are successfully performed on embryos
Cryopreservation survival rate	(Number of embryos surviving thawing/total number of embryos thawed) × 100	Measures the percentage of embryos that survive the freezing and thawing process
Patient satisfaction rate	(Number of satisfied patients/total number of patients surveyed) × 100	Measures overall satisfaction of patients with the services provided in the ART lab

that evaluates the effectiveness of a technique and individual efforts by comparing the number of fertilised oocytes. Parameters like cleavage rate and blastocyst formation rate are also monitored to understand embryonic growth and factors leading to pregnancies. Another vital metric is the success rate of PGT, which indicates the precision of biopsy techniques and the efficiency of testing procedures.

Critical KPIs encompass the survival rate of embryos and the count of cryopreserved oocytes or embryos both per patient and cumulatively across multiple cycles.

12.6 Management KPIs

The rate at which cycles are cancelled, known as the cycle cancellation rate (CCR), is a metric that evaluates how well patients are managed and gives insight into the success of treatments. Another crucial indicator is the time-to-pregnancy (TTP). This metric not only shows how effective treatment strategies are but also directly measures patient satisfaction. It contributes to an understanding of the patient experience.

Turnaround time (TAT) is a measure of the clinic's efficiency. It calculates the duration from when an ART cycle starts until it is completed or terminated. At the same time, analysing retention and dropout rates gives valuable insights into how well the clinic performs. These rates help determine how successful labs are in creating a comfortable environment for patients and retaining them after unsuccessful cycles.

Together, these KPIs provide a view of the clinic's efficiency, patient satisfaction, and overall effectiveness in fertility treatment strategies. They play a role in improving practices, managing quality, and advancing knowledge within the field of fertility treatment.

12.7 Measurement and Tracking of KPIs

Establishing uniform guidelines and optimal practices, such as those outlined in the Istanbul Consensus Workshop on Embryo Assessment, is essential to standardising and controlling the quality of KPI measurement in ART. These guidelines offer a universal standard for grading and assessing embryos. Implementing external quality assessment programmes and proficiency evaluations is vital to confirming laboratories' compliance with established standards. These initiatives are essential in determining the laboratory's aptitude and consistency in generating reliable and accurate outcomes.

12.8 Challenges and Solutions Focusing on ART Lab KPIs

Inconsistent measurement: There can be variability in measuring and reporting KPIs, making comparing data across different cycles or laboratories challenging.

Solution: Achieving this objective involves implementing protocols and guidelines for laboratory procedures for training staff members on measurement techniques.

High cost of technology: Some technologies used to measure KPIs in ART labs, such as time-lapse imaging, may be expensive to implement and maintain.

Solution: ART labs explore cost-effective alternatives for measuring KPIs, including traditional microscopy and manual embryo scoring.

Lack of skilled staff: Skilled embryologists and lab technicians are required to measure KPIs accurately, but more qualified personnel are often lacking.

Solution: Labs may explore the adoption of automated semen analysis and related technologies to complement the expertise of their staff, resulting in improved efficiency and accuracy in laboratory operations.

Ethical considerations: Using technology to measure KPIs may generate ethical concerns regarding using embryos in research.

Solution: We must seek informed consent from patients before using their embryos for research.

Data access: It can be quite challenging to gather data for measuring performance indicators due to limited access to patient information.

Solution: ART labs can collaborate with healthcare providers to facilitate information exchange. Additionally, there is a proposal to introduce health record systems that would centralise data in a secure and easily accessible manner; this would greatly enhance the availability of data for KPI measurement purposes.

Adverse events: The accuracy of KPI measurements and treatment outcomes may be negatively affected by adverse events during ART procedures

Solution: ART labs need contingency plans to address regular equipment maintenance, strict adherence to lab protocols, and staff training on emergency response procedures.

Patient variability: Patient age and medical history may impact treatment outcomes and KPI measurement accuracy.

Solution: ART labs develop patient selection criteria based on evidence-based guidelines and regularly review and update these criteria based on treatment outcomes.

12.9 Evaluating the Competence of Embryologists: Metrics and Methodologies

Embryologists play a vital role in the successful execution of ART treatments, performing a wide range of responsibilities within ART labs. Their primary duties are handling and preparing gametes for fertilisation and closely monitoring the development of embryos in the laboratory. They also carry out IVF, ICSI, and embryo biopsy. Furthermore, embryologists evaluate embryo quality and select the most suitable embryos for transfer.

Maintaining expertise: Assessing embryologist performance helps confirm their proficiency in conducting ART procedures by confirming they possess the required knowledge, skills, and experience.

Opportunities: The success of ART procedures is directly influenced by the performance of embryologists. By evaluating their performance, ART labs can precisely identify ways to enhance laboratory processes and protocols, ultimately leading to higher success rates and better outcomes for patients.

12.10 Possible Recommendations for ART Professionals and Infertility Clinics

Healthcare professionals and infertility clinics use KPIs to track and assess their performance in providing high-quality care to patients.

Identify KPIs: It is important to determine which KPIs are applicable to the clinic's goals and objectives. For example, factors like success rates, satisfaction, wait times, and costs can be considered.

Define targets: Targets help with monitoring progress and ensure that goals are achieved as intended.

Utilise data analytics: Incorporating data analytics tools enables real-time monitoring of KPIs; this process aids in identifying patterns and gaining insights for making decisions that enhance the clinic's performance.

Communication within the team: It is crucial to communicate the chosen KPIs and targets with the team, along with explaining how their work contributes significantly to achieving these goals. This fosters a sense of accountability and promotes a culture of improvement.

Review and adjust KPIs: Frequent evaluation of KPIs and objectives is essential to maintaining their relevance over time while ensuring they align with the current goals of the clinic.

12.11 KPI Benchmark Value

The KPIs listed in Table 12.2 correspond to essential procedures or stages of embryonic development in ART. For example, the ICSI degeneration rate, the normal fertilisation rate for both IVF and ICSI, and the cleavage rate represent critical measurement points that directly influence fertility treatment's overall success.

TABLE 12.2

KPI Benchmark Values (ESHRE)

Key Performance Indicator	Competency Value	Benchmark Value
ICSI degeneration rate	≤10%	≤5%
ICSI normal fertilisation rate (2PN)	≥65%	≥80%
IVF normal fertilisation rate (2PN)	≥60%	≥75%
Failed fertilisation rate (IVF)		<5%
Cleavage rate	≥95%	≥99%
Day 2 embryo development rate	≥50%	≥80%
Day 3 embryo development rate	≥45%	≥70%
Blastocyst development rate	≥40%	≥60%
Successful biopsy rate	≥90%	≥95%
Cryosurvival rate	≥90%	≥99%
Implantation rate (cleavage stage)	≥25%	≥35%
Implantation rate (blastocyst stage)	≥35%	≥60%

The benchmark values for each of these KPIs serve two key roles.

Quality assurance: These values establish a measurable standard that all fertility clinics should aim to meet or surpass. They are crucial in maintaining high-quality care and treatment across all clinics, ensuring that every patient receives excellent care.

Improvement: The benchmark values act as targets that encourage improvement. By striving to achieve these benchmarks, clinics can optimise their treatment protocols and methodologies, leading to better outcomes for patients. This pushes clinics to evaluate their performance, identify areas for enhancement, and take steps to elevate their practice.

This approach fosters a cycle of quality improvement and sets the stage for improved fertility treatment outcomes. By providing clinics with targets, this framework guides clinics in delivering patient care, constantly refining their practices, and ultimately enhancing the success rates of ART procedures.

CHAPTER 12

SUMMARY

- KPIs are measurements used to evaluate the performance and success of organisations, departments, or individuals.
- ART labs use benchmarking to compare their KPIs to industry standards or best practices, allowing them to detect areas for improvement and make data-driven decisions.
- KPIs are used to assess the effectiveness of changes or improvements made in ART labs, providing insights into the impact of process changes or new technologies.
- KPIs monitor compliance with regulatory standards and accreditation requirements, supporting ongoing quality control and improvement efforts.
- While KPIs are a crucial tool for evaluating ART lab performance, it is crucial to consider their limitations and use them with other evaluation methods to provide a comprehensive view of lab performance.
- The Vienna consensus guidelines provide recommendations for measuring and reporting KPIs in ART clinics.
- Clinical, laboratory, and management KPIs are developed to track infertility evaluation and management performance.
- Accurate and reliable data collection is vital for measuring and tracking KPIs.
- Standardising data collection and data accuracy are challenges in measuring and tracking ART lab KPIs.
- KPIs are used to evaluate the competence of embryologists in ART labs.
- Metrics for evaluating embryologist competence are embryo development, implantation, and pregnancy rates.
- Regular assessments, peer review, and competency-based training programmes are methodologies for evaluating embryologist competence.
- KPI calculations vary based on the specific metric being evaluated.
- Standard KPI calculations in ART labs are pregnancy rates, live birth rates, and time-to-pregnancy.

13

ART Lab Witnessing Systems

In the intricate environment of the ART lab, every procedure's accuracy is of paramount importance. The witnessing system serves as an essential component, offering a critical layer of quality control to ensure precision and reliability. The process leverages two key roles: 1) the performer who conducts the ART procedure and 2) the witness, a vigilant observer who authenticates each step without direct participation in the procedure itself. This dual-control approach minimises errors, ensuring safety and efficacy.

The witness primarily validates the correlation between the patient and the treatment while affirming the correct use of medications and equipment, thereby ensuring that standardised protocols are maintained. Simultaneously, the performer implements the ART procedure, adhering to set protocols and maintaining clear communication with the witness. This cooperation promotes accountability and seamless procedural execution.

The significance of witnessing an ART lab is manifold. It helps prevent potential errors and mix-ups, thereby averting catastrophic outcomes for patients and their families. It reinforces the accuracy and consistency of procedures, bolstering patient safety by confirming the suitability of the medications and equipment used. Witnessing also enhances procedure transparency, increasing patient trust and confidence in the process.

Different types of witnessing include technical, procedural, and interpretative witnessing. In technical witnessing, the witness ensures that all equipment is utilised correctly and calibrated and that samples are handled appropriately. They also carry out quality control checks to swiftly identify and rectify any discrepancies.

Procedural witnessing entails the witness confirming the correct identification and treatment of patients. This role requires careful tracking and verification of samples along with stringent adherence to labelling and documentation standards, thereby maintaining procedural integrity.

Interpretative witnessing involves the witness validating the precision and reliability of testing outcomes. They also ensure that established quality control standards are met for all procedures and that any errors identified are promptly rectified. Each type of witnessing is essential in its own way, contributing to the overall quality and safety of procedures in the ART lab.

13.1 Manual Witnessing System

Manual witnessing involves assigning two witnesses who are laboratory technicians or embryologists with the expertise to oversee and validate the handling of gametes and embryos throughout the entire process.

The witnesses are responsible for steps including preparation, egg fertilisation, embryo culture, and freezing. At the end of each procedure, these witnesses confirm the procedure's

DOI: 10.1201/9781032622736-13

accuracy by signing a document. This document is then stored in the clinic's records as a point of reference for any disputes or investigations regarding procedures.

Manual witnessing goes beyond being a formality; it serves as a mechanism to maintain the quality and precision of ART procedures. Despite advancements, it remains a practised approach in ART labs worldwide (Tables 13.1 and 13.2).

TABLE 13.1

Model 1: Witnessing Checklist—Seminology

ABC Fertility Centre			
Witnessing checklist—Seminology			
Female name:	Date of birth:	Hospital ID	
Male name:	Date of birth:	Date:	
Clinical/lab activity	**Practitioner**	**Witness**	**Time**
Patient verification check			
Semen sample ID check			
Sperm preparation tube 1 check			
Sperm preparation tube 2 check			
Overlay check			
Insemination check			
Sperm freezing vial ID check			
Sperm storage location			
Removal of sperm from storage ID check			
Documentation completion check			

TABLE 13.2

Model 2—Embryology Procedure: Witness Checklist

ABC Fertility Centre				
Female Name:	Date of birth:	Hospital ID:		
Male Name:	Date of birth:	Date:		
Activity	Embryologist	Witness	Instructions	Comments
OOCYTE PICK UP				
Patient name and ID verification			Oral cross-check between practitioner and witness	
Egg collection and incubation dish label check				
DENUDATION CHECK				
Hylase dish prepared at least one hour prior to use			Oral cross-check between practitioner and witness	
Pre-ICSI dish label check				
ICSI/INSEMINATION CHECK				
ICSI dish prepared at least two hours prior				
ICSI stage check				
ICSI dish label check while adding sperm			Oral cross-check between practitioner and witness	
Sperm ID check				
Needles aligned and tested				
Sperm addition/IVF/ICSI dish				
Post-ICSI dish label check				

(Continued)

TABLE 13.2 *(Continued)*

Model 2—Embryology Procedure: Witness Checklist

ABC Fertility Centre		
Female Name:	Date of birth:	Hospital ID:
Male Name:	Date of birth:	Date:
PN CHECK AND DAY 2 EMBRYO CHECK		
IVF dish to cleavage dish		
Check stage temperature		Oral cross-check between
Check zygote dish label		practitioner and witness
ZYGOTE DISH TO DAY 3 DISH		
Zygote dish label check		Oral cross-check between
Day 3 dish label check		practitioner and witness
DAY 3 DISH TO BLASTOCYST DISH		
Day 3 dish label check		Oral cross-check between
Day 5 dish label check		practitioner and witness
EMBRYO TRANSFER DISH		
Embryo dish label check		Oral cross-check between
Embryo transfer dish label check		practitioner and witness
EMBRYO FREEZING DISH		
Check details on embryo dish		Oral cross-check between
Check details on goblet, cryolock, cryocan, and cryovial		practitioner and witness

13.2 Electronic Witnessing

Electronic witnessing is a modern and efficient method for ensuring the safety and quality of procedures performed in ART labs. Moreover, ART procedures encompass complex laboratory techniques and the handling of delicate biological samples, which are prone to errors and mishandling.

Therefore, QC measures are crucial in ART labs to ensure that the samples are handled accurately, efficiently, and safely. Witnessing is a quality control measure that entails documenting every step of the ART process and confirming the identity of each sample. Traditionally, ART laboratories have employed manual witnessing, but a sophisticated automated method is now available with the advent of electronic witnessing. Electronic witnessing has become an indispensable instrument for ensuring the quality and safety of ART procedures, and its use is anticipated to rise in the years ahead.

13.3 Types of Electronic Witnessing Systems

Radio frequency identification (RFID) technology: RFID tags contain a unique code that RFID readers scan. The readers use radio waves to communicate with the tags and gather information on their location and status.

RFID readers can be fixed, laptop, or mobile. Fixed readers are typically installed in sample storage areas or workstations, while mobile readers are handheld or mounted on carts and used to read tags in different locations. The choice of reader will depend on the specific needs of the ART lab and the procedures being performed.

RFID tags are attached to instruments and equipment, allowing real-time tracking and scheduling maintenance. RFID tags can also be attached to media and consumables, helping to confirm that the correct items are used for each procedure.

13.3.1 Advantages of RFID

RFID technology makes tracking samples, equipment, and personnel reliable and reduces the chances of errors. This leads to high-quality procedures in the lab. In addition to enhancing accuracy, RFID systems also save time. They automate the tracking process, allowing staff to increase productivity and focus on specific tasks. Regarding security, RFID systems are highly beneficial, acting as a deterrent against access to equipment and samples and thus improving lab security. Finally, the integration capabilities of RFID systems are impressive. These systems can seamlessly integrate with laboratory information management systems (LIMS), promoting a workflow without interruptions.

13.3.2 Limitations of the RFID System

- Cost: RFID systems are expensive to implement and maintain, particularly for smaller labs.
- Complexity: RFID may be complex to set up and require technical expertise.
- Interference: They are subject to interference from other electronic devices and materials, which affects their accuracy.

13.3.3 Barcode Technology

Barcodes contain ID numbers, sample numbers, and dates. Staff should be provided with barcode scanners so that they can easily read the barcodes on samples and containers.

Barcode systems offer advantages for smaller laboratories. One key benefit is their cost-effectiveness. Setting up a barcode system requires effort, and staff need training to use it effectively. Accuracy is also an advantage of barcode systems since they enable the tracking of samples, equipment, and personnel. Furthermore, barcode systems seamlessly integrate into the lab's workflow. Staff members can easily verify materials at each step, ensuring the correct usage of materials and adherence to protocols.

13.3.4 Limitations of the Barcode System

- The amount of information that can be stored in barcodes is limited, and in some cases it may need to be updated to meet tracking requirements.
- Barcodes need to be scanned in proximity to the reader, which can be inconvenient in certain situations.
- Barcode labels may be damaged over time, leading to readability issues.

13.3.5 Biometric Identification

Biometrics rely on unique attributes such as fingerprints or retinal patterns to authenticate an individual's identity. Within an ART lab environment, biometric systems ensure that authorised personnel carry out each step of the procedures. Prior to granting access to equipment or samples, individuals' biometric data is recorded in a database and utilised for identity verification purposes.

Biometric systems offer a range of benefits, beginning with improved security. By allowing authorised personnel to access equipment and samples, biometric systems help maintain a level of security within the laboratory. This precision enhances the integrity of the laboratory's procedures and processes. Another notable advantage is convenience. Biometric systems eliminate the need for staff members to carry ID cards or remember passwords, making identification and access control seamless and hassle-free. Therefore, incorporating biometrics strengthens lab security and accuracy and adds convenience to daily operations for lab personnel.

13.3.6 Limitations of the Biometric System

- Privacy concerns: Some individuals may be concerned about their privacy regarding the collection and storage of biometric data.
- Technical issues: Technical difficulties, like low image quality or system failures, may affect biometric systems.

13.4 Video Monitoring

It is important to ensure that the positioning of cameras throughout the lab captures all steps and procedures. Additionally, videos should record and securely store all video footage for a period of time, per rules and regulations. In cases where disputes or questions arise regarding sample or embryo handling, recorded video footage can serve as evidence. This helps clarify situations, resolve misunderstandings, and address concerns.

13.5 Implementation of Electronic Witnessing

Security and confidentiality: It is crucial to implement witnessing in a way that ensures information protection and compliance with privacy laws and regulations.

Technical infrastructure: Selecting the technology for ART labs is vital. Factors such as lab size, procedure complexity, and desired accuracy and reliability should be considered when creating requirements. Electronic witnessing may involve utilising laptops or tablets as video conferencing platforms and ensuring an Internet connection.

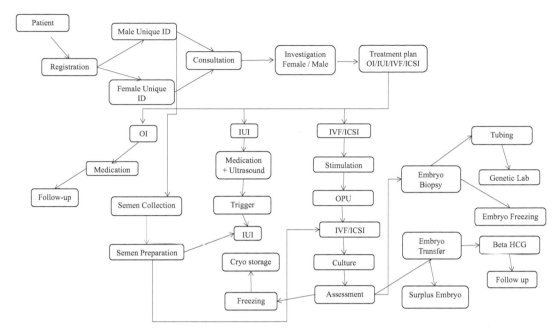

FIGURE 13.1
Flowchart of ART lab workflow and checkpoints.

SOP: Developing a protocol for employing electronic witnessing is essential. Additionally, providing training to all personnel involved in the process is equally crucial. Ensuring that all required hardware and software are in place and functioning properly is also part of this SOP.

Training and support: It is imperative that the staff at the ART lab receive training on electronic witnessing techniques as well as be familiarised with the supporting technology.

13.6 Applications of Electronic Witnessing

Patient identification and sample labelling: Each patient's files and samples (sperm, eggs, and embryos) are assigned barcodes or RFID tags to ensure identification and to reduce the risk of mix-ups. During each step of the process, the barcodes or RFID tags are scanned to confirm that the correct patient samples are being used.

Sperm preparation: During the sperm washing and preparation steps, barcode scanning or RFID tagging is employed to track the sperm samples. This allows for documentation of parameters such as sperm concentration, motility, and other relevant factors to maintain precise records.

Oocyte retrieval: Barcodes or RFID tags are used to track both follicular fluid and oocytes during the retrieval process.

IVF or ICSI: Electronic witnessing is utilised to verify that the correct sperm and egg samples are combined during IVF or ICSI procedures.

Embryo culture and assessment: Culture dishes or wells containing embryos are labelled with barcodes or RFID tags to ensure proper tracking throughout the culture period. Electronic documentation is maintained for embryo development, grading, and any observations made during this time.

Cryopreservation: To preserve and store embryos, it is recommended to use barcodes or RFID tags on cryovials or straws. These tags ensure tracking of stored embryos, while electronic documentation helps maintain records and simplifies future searches within the storage system.

QC: These systems help identify trends, potential issues, and areas for improvement. Additionally, implementing audit trails allows tracking of any changes made to records, including who made the change, when it was made, and what was changed.

Electronic witnessing brings a boost to efficiency in intricate procedures, as it is faster and more effective than manual witnessing. It reduces the time spent on paperwork and allows for real-time verification of each step in the process. Incorporating RFID tags, barcodes, and biometrics into witnessing greatly improves accuracy by minimising errors and inconsistencies. This ensures the correct handling of samples and equipment at every stage. Additionally, electronic witnessing seamlessly integrates with laboratory systems and software, making data transfer smooth and enhancing efficiency.

Electronic witnessing provides a detailed account of the process, which proves invaluable for audits and quality control purposes. This feature simplifies sample tracking and equipment management and quickly identifies any discrepancies or errors, further solidifying its significance in laboratory practices.

13.7 Limitations of Electronic Witnessing

Cost: Implementing witnessing requires technology and resources, which can be financially burdensome for certain laboratories.

Complexity: The integration and maintenance of electronic witnessing may pose challenges compared to manual witnessing. It necessitates planning and coordination to effectively incorporate equipment and procedures into the system.

System failures: Electronic witnessing systems are susceptible to equipment malfunctions or system crashes. These issues have the potential to disrupt laboratory operations.

13.8 The Future of Electronic Witnessing

The anticipated technological advancements and stricter regulatory standards forecast a significant expansion in the use of electronic witnessing in ART labs. Numerous potential evolutions within this technology could redefine the future landscape of electronic witnessing.

Blockchain technology: Blockchain technology is a distributed ledger system used to create a tamper-proof record of transactions. In ART labs, blockchain technology could create an immutable record of sample movement and testing results. This technology could improve the security and reliability of electronic witness systems.

Artificial intelligence: AI technology could improve the accuracy and efficiency of electronic witnessing systems. AI algorithms are used, for instance, to identify potential errors or anomalies in sample tracking data, alerting lab personnel to potential problems before they become significant.

Internet of Things (IoT): Utilising Internet of Things (IoT) technology, which leverages sensors to oversee parameters like location and temperature, can trace samples and equipment in real time, and this potential enhancement can amplify the precision and efficiency of electronic witnessing systems, thereby diminishing the likelihood of mistakes and bolstering the overall quality of the testing process

Wearable technology: The movement of lab personnel and samples could be monitored using wearable technology, such as smartwatches or RFID identifiers. This technology could improve the accuracy of electronic witnessing systems by ensuring that each sample is correctly tracked and recorded.

Cloud computing: Cloud-based systems have the potential to facilitate the storage and analysis of vast amounts of data generated by electronic witness systems. If implemented, a cloud computing strategy can improve the effectiveness and scalability of said systems. This would allow laboratories to manage more samples and reduce their chance of errors.

The choice of which system to use will depend on the needs and resources of the lab. It is important to consider factors such as cost, accuracy, convenience, and integration when deciding on a witnessing system.

Looking ahead, the future of witnessing appears promising. With advancements in technologies like blockchain and AI, there is potential for levels of accuracy, security, and efficiency. However, it is crucial to remember that the effectiveness of witnessing systems relies heavily on the individuals operating them. Proper training and consistent monitoring of system performance are essential to ensuring that electronic witnessing remains accurate and effective in ART laboratories.

CHAPTER 13

SUMMARY

- Implementing witnessing systems within IVF laboratories guarantees the accurate identification of samples, prevents potential mix-ups, and upholds quality control standards.

- There are two main types of witnessing: manual witnessing and electronic witnessing.

- Manual witnessing involves a second person physically verifying sample credentials and handling them during critical procedures.

- Manual witnessing is effective but subject to human error and may be time consuming.

- Electronic witnessing uses technology to track, verify, and document sample identification and handling, reducing human error.

- Types of electronic witnessing systems consist of barcode scanners, RFID tags, and specialised software and hardware solutions.

- Implementing electronic witnessing requires selecting an appropriate system, integrating it into workflows, and training staff.

- The benefits of electronic witnessing consist of improved accuracy, increased efficiency, enhanced traceability, and a reduced risk of errors.

- Limitations of electronic witnessing include high initial costs, potential technological failures, and ongoing maintenance and support needs.

- The potential developments in electronic witnessing may encompass technological advancements, incorporation with other laboratory systems, and broader implementation in IVF labs.

14

Case Studies

14.1 Examples of Successful Quality Control Practices

To uphold standards, it is crucial to incorporate QMS. An exemplary QMS practice in an ART lab involves integrating a programme that includes staff training, competency assessments, and participation in external quality assurance initiatives. This multi-faceted approach ensures that all lab personnel are well trained and regularly evaluated for their competence, thus maintaining excellence over time (Figure 14.1).

Implementing such a programme can lead to improvements across numerous areas within an ART lab. It enhances efficiency, reliability, and the success of procedures performed. Moreover, it helps minimise errors, improve outcomes, and ensure compliance with regulations and standards. In essence, the systematic application of a QMS significantly contributes to the performance and reputation of an ART lab; it is truly indispensable.

Recognising the importance of quality and safety in ART clinics, the ESHRE has devoted efforts towards developing guidelines for quality management in these clinics. These guidelines include recommendations on laboratory design, equipment usage, and SOPs.

Additionally, the College of American Pathologists offers accreditation programmes along with proficiency testing programmes specifically designed for ART labs. These programmes offer evaluations of quality from various sources as well as providing opportunities for laboratories to assess their performance compared to other labs and identify areas for improvement.

As an example, the ART laboratory at the University of California, San Francisco (UCSF) implemented a programme to enhance the consistency and excellence of embryo transfer procedures. This involved staff training, competency assessments, and the integration of time-lapse imaging to monitor embryo development and transfer. The outcomes of this programme were impressive, with improvements in implantation and live birth rates.

Recognising the importance of maintaining high quality service standards, the Fertility Centre of Las Vegas implemented a programme that included operating procedures, regular equipment maintenance, ongoing staff education, and active participation in quality assurance initiatives.

Additionally, the Colorado Centre for Reproductive Medicine (CCRM) has enacted a quality control protocol aimed at standardising procedures and ensuring reliable test results. This programme has produced outcomes that include increases in conception rates and a reduction in the number of embryos required per reproductive cycle. CCRM's commitment to improving fertility outcomes and providing care is evident through their execution of this quality assurance initiative.

Reproductive Medicine Associates of New Jersey (RMANJ) introduced a quality control initiative that incorporated a database to monitor aspects of ART procedures such as

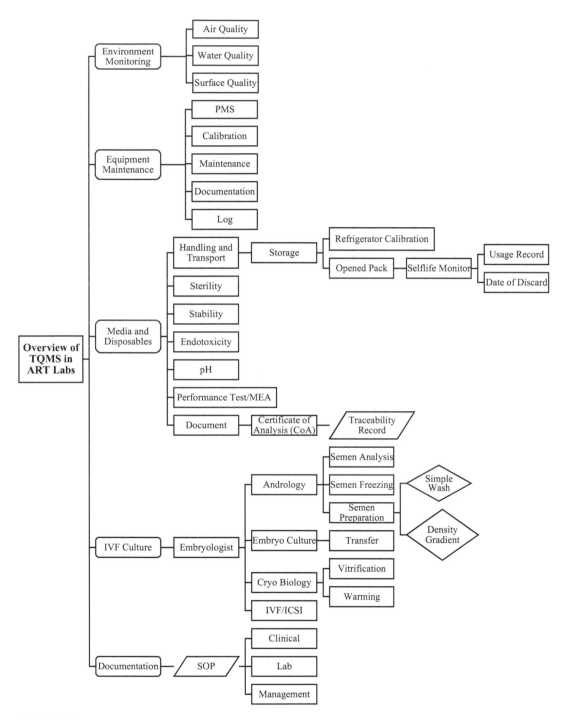

FIGURE 14.1
Overview of TQMS in ART labs.

patient information, laboratory processes, and results. This system aided in enhancing the precision and uniformity of data collection, consequently resulting in advancements in ART outcomes.

14.2 Real-World Examples of QC in ART Labs

In recent years, there have been reports about mistakes occurring in ART clinics worldwide during IVF procedures. These unfortunate incidents emphasise the importance of quality control and adherence to best practices in managing IVF treatments. For example, during the mid-2010s, couples discovered that implanted embryos were not genetically related to them.

In the early 2020s, incidents involving mix-ups with sperm came to light. This also led to babies being born without any connection to their intended fathers. In some instances, these mix-ups were only discovered after birth, resulting in emotional upheaval for the affected families.

An interesting case from the 2000s involved a couple who expected twins through IVF but were surprised when their babies displayed different ethnic characteristics than themselves. This indicated a mix-up of material during the IVF process

These events are a reminder of how important it is for fertility clinics to have quality control measures in place. Errors can have an impact on families, raising concerns about the protocols used to ensure accurate handling and identification of genetic material in these clinics.

14.3 Preventing Mix-Ups

Mix-ups and witnessing failure are serious errors that occur in ART labs, requiring different approaches to prevention and mitigation.

There is a possibility of mix-ups occurring due to mishandling of samples or during the embryo transfer process. For instance, there could be errors of using samples meant for one patient on another or unintentionally mixing up samples from patients. Confusion may also arise from communication and documentation mistakes in certain situations. To prevent these mix-ups, it is important to ensure that all patient samples are properly labelled, strict adherence to operating procedures is followed, and regular staff training on handling and labelling protocols is conducted. Some labs also use systems to verify identities and ensure that the correct samples are used.

Witnessing failure refers to when the system designed to guarantee the use of gametes, embryos, or samples for each patient breaks down. This can occur due to sample labelling or staff members not following procedures.

To prevent witnessing failures in ART labs, it is crucial to establish a witnessing system. This involves implementing procedures that accurately verify identities, carefully labelling all samples with identifiers, and diligently tracking sample movement throughout the lab.

The implementation of witnessing systems can provide a layer of protection, minimising the chances of mistakes and offering an added level of verification.

It is essential for ART laboratories to have protocols in place to address incidents where mix-ups or witnessing failures occur. These protocols should involve promptly informing both patients and their medical practitioners about the error, providing counselling and support to those affected, and conducting a review of existing lab procedures to prevent errors.

Mix-ups in IVF procedures have led to distress and legal disputes for families worldwide. The examples mentioned emphasise the importance of having quality assurance measures and transparency in fertility clinics to minimise the possibility of such errors. Furthermore, these incidents highlight the necessity for enhanced support services and counselling for individuals impacted by IVF errors, as well as a robust legal framework to handle the consequences of such mistakes.

CHAPTER 14

SUMMARY

- Successful quality control practices in ART labs include staff training, competency assessment, and participation in external quality assurance programmes.
- Several fertility clinics have implemented quality control programmes, leading to increased pregnancy rates and improved procedures.
- Real-world mix-ups in ART labs have caused emotional distress and legal battles for affected families.
- Proper quality control, regulation, and transparency are essential in fertility clinics to minimise the risk of errors.
- ART labs must implement strict protocols and witnessing systems to prevent mix-ups and witness failures.
- The fertility industry should continuously work on improving procedures and protocols.
- It is imperative to offer emotional assistance and counselling services to individuals affected by errors in IVF labs.
- A robust legal framework is needed to address the consequences of IVF mistakes.
- Regular reviews and updates to standard operating procedures can ensure they align with current best practices and guidelines from professional organisations.
- Centres should provide ongoing education and training opportunities for ART lab staff to enhance skills and remain current with new developments in the field.
- Centres should establish a transparent and efficient system for reporting and addressing errors or incidents in ART labs to facilitate learning and continuous improvement.
- Centres should encourage patient involvement and communication throughout the ART process to confirm patients are well-informed and comfortable with the procedures.
- Centres should monitor and evaluate the effectiveness of implemented quality control practices and make adjustments to optimise patient outcomes.

15

Emerging Trends and Best Practices: New Technologies in QC

Advancements in ART laboratories have brought improvements to QC. These innovations aim to enhance accuracy, safety, and efficiency in ART procedures, ultimately improving the level of healthcare provided to patients.

One advanced approach used for sperm evaluation is CASA. Compared to other techniques, CASA methods provide accurate assessments of sperm samples. By offering real-time assessment of sperm parameters, CASA technology delivers data for analysis.

Time-lapse imaging technology captures the growth and division patterns of embryos, providing insights for selecting embryos and increasing the chances of implantation.

The advent of PGT has revolutionised embryonic assessment for abnormalities and genetic mutations. Modern PGT techniques, like next-generation sequencing (NGS) and array genomic hybridisation (aCGI I), offer enhanced accuracy and comprehensive genetic testing capabilities, reducing the risk of genetic disorders or miscarriage.

Non-invasive preimplantation genetic testing (niPGT) involves extracting material from the culture medium surrounding the embryo instead of performing an invasive biopsy on the embryo itself. This approach minimises invasiveness while still providing information (Figure 15.1).

Various noninvasive methods exist to assess the quality and viability of embryos, including time lapse imaging, metabolomics, and proteomics. Unlike other procedures, these methods provide information about embryo development, cell division patterns, and metabolic profiles without causing any damage.

Digital quality control systems like laboratory notebooks and laboratory information management systems have improved data management and accuracy in documentation. They help reduce the likelihood of errors or omissions in ART laboratories.

The concept of patient-centred care has gained prominence in ART treatments. It emphasises approaches that cater to patients' needs and preferences. This comprehensive approach focuses not only on procedures but also provides emotional support through counselling, support groups, and complementary therapies.

Standardised quality indicators have been developed to assess the quality of ART procedures and outcomes. These indicators promote consistency and reliability across clinics and countries, enabling comparisons and benchmarking.

Single-cell RNA sequencing (scRNA seq) is a technique that provides detailed information about gene expression and cell differentiation during embryo development. These techniques offer insights into mechanisms and potential biomarkers for selecting embryos.

DOI: 10.1201/9781032622736-15

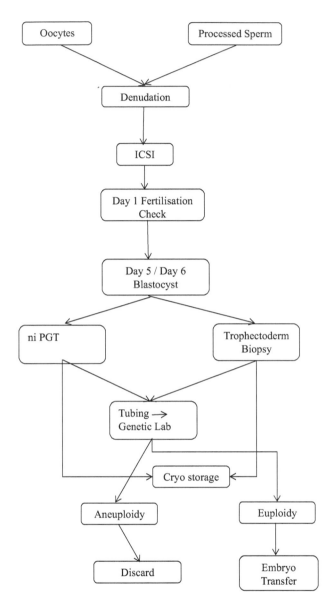

FIGURE 15.1
Overview of non-invasive PGT/trophectoderm (TE) biopsy.

15.1 ART Lab Automation

Automation, including the use of robots, is revolutionising ART. Increasingly common in ART laboratories, robotic systems are now being utilised in procedures to improve efficiency and precision throughout the ART process.

While preparing sperm, robots can automate the selection and preparation steps. They can isolate high-quality sperm based on predetermined criteria, eliminating the need for identification, reducing the risk of human error, and ensuring consistent and reliable outcomes.

During oocyte retrieval, robotic systems can assist by positioning the needle used to collect follicles. They can be programmed to calculate the angle and depth for needle insertion, which increases procedure accuracy while minimising harm to surrounding tissues.

In ICSI, a procedure that requires precision, robots offer significant advantages. They provide control and stability, enabling the immobilisation and injection of a single sperm into an oocyte. Robotic systems can also assist in monitoring the injection process to ensure delivery of the sperm while minimising any risk of damage to the oocyte.

Robotic automation is also utilised in embryo culture, where maintaining controlled and consistent conditions is vital for embryo development.

Robots in incubators can maintain optimal conditions, ensuring appropriate temperature, humidity, and gas concentrations; this reduces the need for monitoring and handling embryos, minimising disturbances and improving the chances of embryo growth.

The use of robotics in ART labs has advantages. Automation decreases reliance on labour, freeing up embryologists to focus on complex tasks. It enhances consistency and precision, since robotic systems can perform tasks without variation or errors. This standardisation improves the reliability and reproducibility of ART procedures, leading to improved patient outcomes.

Moreover, automation streamlines processes in ART labs by optimising workflow and reducing procedure times. Integrating robotics with intelligence and time-lapse imaging allows data integration and analysis, further enhancing the efficiency and accuracy of ART procedures.

While robotic automation offers several benefits, in ART labs it is important to note that human expertise and oversight remain crucial. Embryologists and clinicians play key roles in decision-making processes, result interpretation, and overall patient care. Robots serve as tools that support their expertise by executing tasks consistently.

15.2 Best Practices for Quality Control

To ensure that patient care in ART labs is at its best, it is important to follow guidelines for quality control. There are several elements that contribute to maintaining high standards of quality in ART laboratories.

One crucial aspect is the implementation and strict adherence to SOPs across all ART procedures. SOPs provide a reproducible framework for practices such as handling gametes and embryos, maintaining culture conditions, cryopreservation, and quality assessment. Following SOPs helps ensure accuracy, reliability, and uniformity in the laboratory's operations.

Regular maintenance and calibration of equipment are also essential to obtaining reliable test results. By following scheduled maintenance protocols and ensuring calibration, ART labs can minimise the risk of malfunctions while preserving the integrity of their processes.

Continuous training and competency assessments for staff members are paramount to maintaining quality in ART labs. Ongoing education keeps lab personnel up to date with developments and new techniques in medicine, enabling them to provide optimal care to patients. Regular competency assessments help identify areas for improvement while ensuring that all team members are proficient in their roles.

Internal and external quality assurance programmes are central to ART labs. These programmes facilitate performance monitoring, identify areas that need improvement, and allow benchmarking against industry standards.

Quality assurance activities within a laboratory can encompass proficiency testing, internal audits, and routine process evaluations. Independent assessments through proficiency testing and certification play a role in evaluating the lab's performance while also highlighting areas for growth and enhancement.

Maintaining documentation and meticulous record-keeping are crucial for quality control in ART labs. Accurate and comprehensive records enable traceability, identify patterns and trends, and offer insights for refining processes. It is imperative for ART labs to adhere to guidelines and ensure compliance with industry standards that are relevant to their operations. By staying up to date on regulations and guidelines, ART labs can ensure their practices align with requirements. Regular internal audits and external inspections serve as tools to identify any areas of non-compliance promptly so that corrective actions can be taken.

SAFETY MEASURES AND BEST PRACTICES PROTOCOLS IN ART LABORATORIES

Quality assurance is the basis for a laboratory service to deliver reliable services to users, clinicians, and patients. Quality control is a set of tools to determine whether assessments themselves deliver reliable results.

The examination of semen, a complex process that is difficult to standardise, can lead to discrepancies, creating potential for variations in outcomes.

- Protective handling: Bodily fluids, particularly semen, may contain infectious agents. Thus, they should be handled and disposed of carefully.
- Vaccination: Laboratory personnel working with human samples should be vaccinated against hepatitis B.
- Lab conduct: Activities such as eating, drinking, smoking, and applying cosmetics are prohibited in the lab to maintain a sterile environment.
- Safe pipetting: Pipetting should be performed using mechanical devices only; pipetting by mouth is not allowed.
- Lab attire: Staff should wear lab coats or gowns in the lab and remove them when leaving.
- Glove use: Disposable gloves (rubber, latex, or vinyl, without powder) should be worn when handling fresh or frozen semen, seminal plasma, or other biological samples. Moreover, these should be discarded when leaving the lab, and they should not be reused.
- Hand washing: Hands should be washed regularly, especially before leaving the lab, after handling samples, and after removing lab attire and gloves.

- Safe handling of sharps: Care should be taken to prevent injuries from sharp objects that may be contaminated with semen. Contact between semen and open skin, wounds, or abrasions should be avoided.
- Biomedical waste management: Biomedical waste should be segregated at the source into the appropriate color-coded bags or containers and should be handled, treated, and disposed of according to local regulations. Special care should be taken with sharps, infectious waste, and cytotoxic waste.
- Use of protective gear: Protective goggles, insulated gloves, and closed shoes should be worn when handling hazardous materials, such as liquid nitrogen.
- Workspace cleaning: The workspace should be cleaned daily with disinfectant and then rinsed with water.
- Safety training: Regular safety training should be conducted to ensure staff are familiar with all safety protocols.
- Incident reporting: Any accidents, spills, or injuries should be immediately reported to the laboratory supervisor.

15.3 Software for TQMS

To effectively manage quality control in fertility clinic chains, there are several software options available. These software solutions offer a range of benefits, such as consolidating information, organising appointment schedules, and handling billing processes. They utilise algorithms and machine learning to analyse data, generate insights, and support decision-making based on evidence. These solutions prioritise record-keeping to ensure traceability and minimise errors. Additionally, they provide modules for quality management, staff training, and document control. Operating on cloud-based systems allows for real-time updates, appointment tracking, and seamless communication between clinics, resulting in improved efficiency. Moreover, these platforms can seamlessly integrate with tools and systems to cater to clinics of different sizes while offering a centralised platform for data management and interpretation. It is important to note that these software solutions strictly adhere to healthcare regulations to ensure compliance within fertility clinics. By promoting collaboration and streamlining workflows across the clinic chain, these solutions help predict outcomes, enhance performance levels, and inform planning efforts.

15.4 AI in Oocyte Prediction

AI algorithms have brought about a transformation in ART labs when it comes to predicting oocyte quality. They offer reliable assessments compared to the subjective and variable manual assessments conducted by experts. By analysing factors such as oocyte morphology, granulation patterns, and nucleus structure, AI models can uncover hidden patterns and characteristics that might escape observers' attention.

15.5 Artificial Intelligence and Machine Learning

ART labs have witnessed advancements in QC thanks to the emergence of AI and ML technologies. These innovative tools have the ability to process high volumes of data produced during ART procedures, enabling real-time monitoring and analysis. By leveraging AI algorithms, we can now identify patterns, predict outcomes, and detect anomalies that might have otherwise gone unnoticed.

15.6 Single-Cell Analysis

The potential for enhancing quality control in ART labs through the analysis of cells is immense. Techniques that focus on analysing cells provide an understanding of embryo quality, genetic abnormalities, and developmental potential. By studying the genetic characteristics of each cell, ART labs can make more informed choices when selecting embryos, which in turn leads to higher success rates and decreases the likelihood of genetic disorders.

15.7 Data Integration and Standardisation

The future of QC in ART labs depends on the integration and standardisation of data. ART labs have the opportunity to create databases that create treatment plans by combining information from different sources, such as patient records, lab results, and treatment outcomes. By standardising methods for collecting, storing, and analysing data, ART labs can ensure consistency and promote collaboration. This ultimately leads to enhanced QC practices and the ability to compare performance benchmarks.

15.8 Artificial Gametes

Artificial gametes, also known as in vitro-derived gametes, are created through laboratory techniques that aim to generate functional sperm or eggs outside the human body. This new technology holds promise for individuals and couples facing infertility or those with genetic disorders who wish to conceive. While artificial gametes are still in the early stages of development, ongoing research is focused on fine-tuning their products and ensuring their safety and efficacy.

15.9 Quality Control Challenges in Artificial Gametes

The development and utilisation of artificial gametes present unique challenges regarding quality control. Ensuring that these synthetic gametes possess the necessary characteristics and functionality is crucial. QC protocols must be established to assess artificial gametes' quality, genetic integrity, and developmental potential. This involves a rigorous evaluation of morphology, genetic stability, epigenetic modifications, and the ability to undergo successful fertilisation and embryonic development.

15.10 Genetic Engineering and Genome Editing

Artificial gametes introduce possibilities for genetic engineering and genome editing techniques. QC processes in ART labs must address the ethical considerations and potential risks associated with manipulating the genetic material of artificial gametes. Stringent quality control measures should be implemented to verify the accuracy, safety, and ethical implications of any genetic modifications introduced.

15.11 Safety and Long-Term Health

QC protocols must encompass comprehensive assessments of potential risks and monitor the long-term outcomes of individuals conceived using these techniques. Longitudinal studies and robust follow-up programmes will be essential to evaluating the health, fertility, and overall well-being of individuals born from ART procedures involving artificial gametes.

15.12 Regulatory Frameworks and Ethical Considerations

The emergence of gametes raises ethical issues that require the creation of strong regulatory frameworks. Quality control procedures should adhere to guidelines to ensure the advancement and utilisation of artificial gametes. Open communication and the active involvement of the public play a role in shaping policies and regulations related to these emerging technologies.

15.13 Improving Quality Control in Donor Gametes

Fertility clinics that offer ART can establish screening measures to ensure the quality of donor gametes. It is crucial to evaluate the health and genetic background of donors to minimise the risk of inherited conditions or infectious diseases. This evaluation process may involve assessments, genetic testing, and screening for infectious diseases to ensure that the donor gametes are safe and suitable.

By prioritising quality control in donor gametes, ART facilities can build trust and confidence among patients. Openly communicating with patients about screening procedures and quality control measures can help alleviate any concerns they may have and promote transparency throughout the process. Providing information about the steps taken to verify the safety and reliability of donor gametes empowers patients to make informed decisions regarding their reproductive options.

CHAPTER 15

SUMMARY

- Emerging technologies and techniques for QC in ART labs include advanced sperm analysis techniques, time-lapse imaging, preimplantation genetic testing, non-invasive monitoring, digital quality control systems, patient-centred care, standardised quality indicators, single-cell analysis, and automation.

- Automation, including robotics, is increasingly prevalent in ART labs, improving efficiency, consistency, and precision in procedures such as sperm preparation, oocyte retrieval, ICSI, and embryo culture.

- Best practices for QC in ART labs involve adhering to standard operating procedures, performing regular equipment maintenance and calibration, providing continuous staff training and competency assessment, participating in internal and external quality assurance programmes, and maintaining proper documentation and record-keeping.

- Artificial gametes offer potential solutions for infertility and genetic disorders, requiring robust QC protocols to assess their quality, genetic stability, developmental potential, and safety implications.

- Ensuring safety and long-term health in ART labs involves comprehensive assessments and follow-up studies for individuals conceived using artificial gametes.

- Regulatory frameworks and ethical considerations are essential in shaping policies surrounding emerging technologies like artificial gametes.

- Improving quality control in donor gametes involves stringent screening protocols, clear communication with patients, and providing detailed information on the safety and reliability of donor gametes.

16

Safety, Recommendations, and Infrastructure

16.1 Safety Measures in ART Labs

ART labs must adhere to safety protocols to minimise the risk of contamination and negative consequences. In ART laboratories, there is a need to handle substances such as cryo-protectants and biological samples, which necessitates the correct utilisation of personal protective equipment and adherence to safe practices.

> **Risk assessment:** Risk assessment is a process that involves identifying and estimating hazards in a workplace, especially in ART labs, where safety is paramount. Handling specimens comes with a risk of exposure to these pathogens. One risk is the possibility of being injured by a needle, which results in exposure to pathogens. In addition to considering the management, storage, and disposal of chemicals, it is important to include measures such as the provision of protective equipment to decrease any potential exposure risks.

Moreover, physical hazards like radiation (UV), electrical hazards, and sharp objects should be evaluated carefully. It is crucial to assess the risks associated with operating equipment while implementing safety protocols that prioritise accident prevention. This entails considering how frequently people may be exposed to these hazards, understanding the consequences of exposure, and assessing the effectiveness. Some examples of control measures may include installing safety cabinets or hoods for processes or developing SOPs that outline safe practices for staff members.

Conducting a risk assessment that considers factors like frequency of exposure, potential consequences, and the efficacy of existing control measures, along with providing thorough training for all staff members, can ensure a safer working environment within ART labs.

Risk assessment should also consider the psychological impact of the work. The work in ART labs can be emotionally demanding and stressful. Therefore, providing mental health support and stress management strategies is also important. Safety assessments must be reviewed to ensure that they remain updated with any modifications in the laboratory setting.

> **Personal protective equipment:** PPE plays a role in safeguarding laboratory staff from exposure to hazardous materials in ART labs. To ensure the safety of the staff, ART labs should carefully evaluate the chemical or physical risks involved and select PPE accordingly. It is important that the chosen PPE effectively protect against these identified hazards and adhere to safety standards.

DOI: 10.1201/9781032622736-16

Aside from providing protection, it is essential to consider the fit and comfort of the PPE. Ill-fitting or uncomfortable PPE may compromise its effectiveness by discouraging usage. Therefore, it is necessary to choose PPE that fits well and allows for movement. Consistently wearing the designated PPE whenever staff members are in contact with materials, performing procedures, or working in risky areas is critical for minimising contamination risks. By following this practice, we can create an environment that reduces the likelihood of exposure incidents. Notably, PPE may become contaminated during use, and prolonged usage can compromise its capabilities. Thus, staff members should be encouraged to change their PPE as needed—especially when transitioning between workstations or handling materials.

Proper training on how to use, handle, and dispose of PPE is necessary for all staff members working in ART labs. This training ensures that everyone understands how to maximise the effectiveness of their equipment while minimising any associated risks.

Hazardous materials: When it comes to disinfectants and cleaning agents, ART labs follow protocols for handling, labelling, and storage.

Liquid nitrogen: The storage area should be equipped with fire extinguishers and emergency eye-wash stations to ensure safety precautions are in place. (See Chapter 10.)

Laboratory waste: In ART labs, hazardous waste requires proper categorisation, handling, and disposal to reduce the risk of exposure to dangerous substances. ART labs should have designated containers for collecting waste that also ensure compatibility with the disposed chemicals. These containers must be labelled appropriately to indicate the nature of the associated hazards.

Safety protocols: To minimise exposure to materials in an ART laboratory, it is important to have safety protocols in place. These guidelines should encompass the upkeep of equipment and incident reporting. ART labs are advised to establish procedures for equipment maintenance that include disinfection protocols.

Proper laboratory design: Designing an ART lab requires careful attention to detail to ensure an effective, secure, and prosperous working environment.

When designing an IVF lab, several key measures should be considered.

Layout and zoning: When designing the layout of ART lab, it is important to consider how the staff, samples, and materials will move within the space. The goal is to create a layout that promotes a workflow of activities and ensures access to each zone. Regularly evaluating and zoning the lab can facilitate identifying areas where improvements can be made. Gathering feedback from staff members and analysing patterns informs adjustments that align with the changing needs of the lab while optimising efficiency (Figure 16.1).

Flooring and surfaces: It is important for workstations to be resistant to chemicals, moisture, and heat. Floors and wall coverings minimise the presence of crevices and joints where dirt and dust build up, resulting in easier cleaning and maintenance while ensuring sterility.

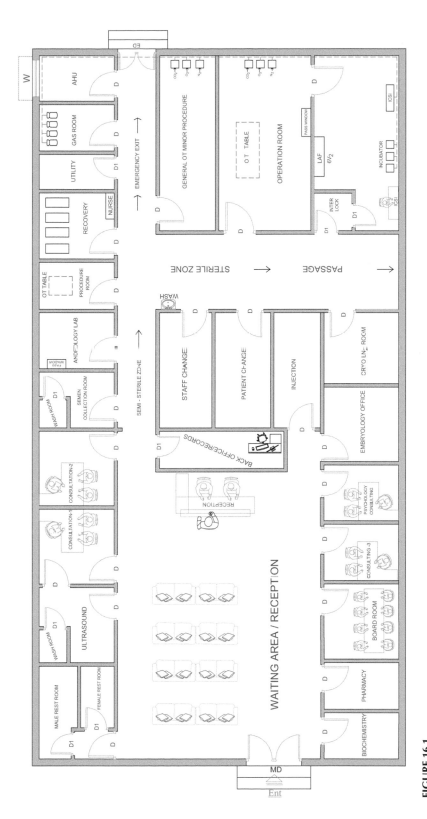

FIGURE 16.1
Layout of a standard ART clinic.

HVAC system: An HVAC system plays a role in maintaining a clean environment for the ART lab by ensuring optimal temperatures, proper humidity levels, and ventilation.

Airlock entry: Airlocks or anterooms should be installed at the entrances to critical areas to minimise the introduction of contaminants. This creates a buffer zone where staff change into protective clothing and footwear before entering the main lab space.

Embryo transfer room: Design a comfortable and private embryo transfer room for patients to undergo the procedure. This room should be adjacent to the embryo culture area to minimise the time and distance between the transfer and the incubators.

Storage and organisation: To maintain a clutter-free and well-organised lab, it is essential to thoughtfully design the storage areas for consumables, reagents, and equipment. Vertical spaces can be efficiently utilised with storage solutions such as cabinets, shelves, and drawers.

Emergency safety features: These should include eye-wash stations, fire extinguishers, and marked emergency exits in case of accidents or emergencies. Additionally, the safety data sheets (SDSs) for all chemicals used in the lab should be within easy reach.

Ergonomics: Proper ergonomic design helps reduce strain on laboratory personnel and enhances productivity, like adjustable chairs, tables, and equipment stands to accommodate the needs of individual users.

Electrical: There should be sufficient electrical outlets and data ports, and using uninterruptible power supply (UPS) systems can protect sensitive equipment during power fluctuations or outages.

Acoustic control: Keeping noise levels in the lab as low as possible is beneficial. A quieter lab environment lowers stress for the staff and, interestingly, the embryos. Research indicates that too much noise might adversely affect embryonic development.

Vibration control: Equipment sensitive to vibrations should be positioned away from potential sources of vibration, like air handling units, elevators, or areas with a lot of foot traffic.

Safety and security: Due to the sensitive nature of their operations, ART facilities must implement stringent security measures to protect patient privacy (Figure 16.2).

Waste management: Designing a waste management system requires careful planning to ensure compliance with local regulations, especially when dealing with hazardous and non-hazardous waste. The system should have dedicated disposal areas for different types of waste that are clearly labelled for correct usage.

Sustainability: As part of the lab design, it would be beneficial to embrace sustainability and use energy-saving lighting options, low-flow water fixtures, and materials that are friendly to the environment.

Cryopreservation room: It is crucial to have ventilation and gas detection systems in place to constantly monitor oxygen levels and promptly detect any nitrogen leaks or oxygen depletion. It is imperative to restrict access to authorised personnel to safeguard samples and confidentiality.

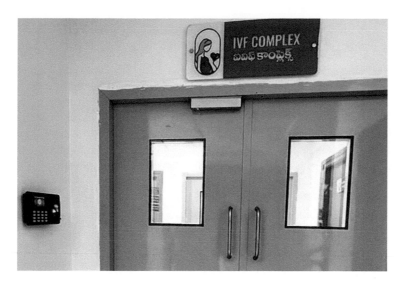

FIGURE 16.2
Photograph showing a fingerprint-reader-based restricted entry to the IVF complex.

Staff facilities: Space within the facility should be allocated for employees to conveniently change clothes, store their belongings, and take breaks. It is important to provide lockers and restrooms for their convenience.

Future expansion: Designing the laboratory flexibly prepares it for growth and possible technological advancements. There should be room for expansion and adaptability to accommodate any developments in ART techniques, equipment, and procedures that may arise.

16.2 Environmental Impact

With increasing attention on sustainability and environmental consciousness, it becomes essential for ART labs, like any other sector, to consider their environmental footprint.

ART laboratories, due to their nature of work, consume significant amounts of energy and produce waste. The high energy consumption is due to the need for constant temperature control and air quality management, which are crucial to maintain the integrity of embryos. In addition, ART labs generate a considerable amount of biomedical waste, including used culture media, plastic consumables, gloves, pipettes, and other lab materials.

Labs could also explore options for recycling non-hazardous waste. Moreover, adopting paperless operations wherever possible, using eco-friendly supplies, and promoting sustainable practices among the staff can further contribute to reducing the lab's environmental footprint.

It is evident that environmental considerations are an integral part of risk management in ART labs. By adopting sustainable practices, these labs can not only reduce their environmental footprint but also improve their efficiency and resilience.

16.3 TQMS for a Chain of Fertility Clinics

Fertility centre chains are especially beneficial for individuals and couples residing in underserved areas with access to fertility services. The advantage of having multiple locations is added convenience and flexibility when it comes to scheduling appointments and procedures.

However, it is important to keep in mind that not all fertility clinics are the same, and the success rates of ART treatments can vary between clinics. It is crucial to research and select a fertility clinic with experienced medical professionals and a proven track record of high success rates.

Advancements: ART advancements encompass aspects such as enhanced embryo assessment, improved stimulation techniques, ICSI allowing embryos to develop further before transfer (blastocyst culture), and the option to freeze embryos for future use. As a result of these progressions, there has been an increase in demand for fertility treatments, leading to the expansion of fertility clinics and chains. However, despite these developments, success rates can still vary depending on factors such as age, overall health, and underlying causes of infertility.

Increase in demand: Infertility is a concern that affects an estimated 10% of couples around the world, and societal attitudes towards infertility have evolved over time, reducing the stigma associated with seeking fertility treatments. The introduction of cryopreservation techniques has also given rise to a trend in ART where individuals seek treatment for fertility issues and consider preserving their fertility. To meet the growing demand, fertility clinics have expanded their services and formed chains to cater to a wider population more efficiently.

Globalisation: With the growth of globalisation, people are increasingly seeking fertility services across borders. This has created a demand for fertility clinics that provide consistent, high-quality care across multiple locations. By expanding their reach across multiple regions, fertility clinic chains can effectively cater to patients who require assistance.

Resource and expertise pooling: Fertility clinic chains can pool their resources and expertise across multiple locations, allowing them to offer a broader range of services and treatments to patients and share knowledge among different clinics.

Economies of scale: Fertility clinics that operate in multiple locations take advantage of economies of scale. By purchasing equipment and supplies in bulk and streamlining processes, they can save costs. These savings are then passed on to patients through cost and accessible treatment options.

16.4 Implementing Total Quality Management Systems in Fertility Clinic Chains

TQMS, also known as a total quality management system, is a strategy aimed at enhancing the quality and effectiveness of a business or organisation.

The following steps can be used to implement a TQMS in a chain of fertility clinics.

Vision and mission: The vision and mission should effectively express the purpose, values, and objectives of the organisation, serving as a compass for decision-making and day-to-day operations at every level.

The vision statement should describe the future state the organisation strives to achieve. The vision for a fertility clinic chain might be 'to become the leading provider of compassionate and effective fertility care, empowering individuals and couples to achieve their dream of building a family'.

The mission statement plays a role in defining the purpose and strategies of an organisation to fulfil its vision. For example, a fertility clinic chain may have a mission statement like this: 'Our aim is to offer inclusive and individualised fertility treatments to both individuals and couples. We utilise cutting-edge technologies and techniques while providing care that is empathetic, compassionate, and respectful'. Objectives should be specific, measurable, and achievable.

Develop a quality policy: A quality policy reflects the organisation's commitment to excellence, outlines its expectations for performance and accountability, and guides decision-making and operations across all levels of the organisation.

16.5 Define Key Performance Indicators

Patient satisfaction is an indispensable KPI, as it measures the level of satisfaction among patients with the clinic's services. (See Chapter 13.)

16.6 Establish a Quality Management Team

Identify team members: The quality management team should include representatives from all levels of the organisation, including senior leadership, clinicians, nurses, lab technicians, and administrative staff.

Each team member needs defined roles and responsibilities for clear accountability. Team members must also undergo training on TQMS principles and methodologies. The development and enforcement of SOPs for critical processes are vital for maintaining consistent operations. The use of technology can enhance operations, reduce errors, and improve patient care. A culture of continuous improvement should be promoted, where employees identify and implement beneficial changes. Moreover, regular audits and reviews of the TQMS ensure its effectiveness and identify areas for refinement.

Implement SOPs: Embracing the use of technology such as EHRs and practice management software can bring about multiple improvements. Electronic records helps streamline operations, reduce errors, and enhance the level of care provided to patients. In addition, fostering a culture of improvement among staff members plays a role in ensuring better patient care and operational efficiency. (See Chapter 11.)

SAMPLE 1: QUALITY POLICY FOR A FERTILITY CLINIC CHAIN

At ABC, we are committed to providing outstanding patient care and services that meet the expectations of our patients and stakeholders. We are dedicated to continuously improving the quality of our services through innovation, education, and ongoing evaluation of our processes and outcomes.

The quality policy is founded on the following principles:

Patient-Centred Care: We prioritise the needs and preferences of our patients and strive to provide care that is compassionate, empathetic, and respectful.

Clinical Excellence: We maintain the highest standards of clinical excellence through ongoing education, training, and quality enhancement initiatives.

Innovation: We embrace new technologies, treatments, and techniques to provide patients with the most advanced and effective care.

Continuous Improvement: We are committed to continuously evaluating our processes by using data to inform our decision-making and improve the quality of our services.

Compliance: We adhere to all applicable laws, regulations, and ethical guidelines and maintain the highest standards of integrity and professionalism in all operations.

16.7 Collaboration

Promoting collaboration across departments and clinics within the fertility clinic chain is key to successful TQMS implementation. This can be achieved through regular meetings, both in person and virtually, to discuss issues and share best practices. Cross-training employees across different departments enhances understanding and collaboration, while a resource-sharing system boosts efficiency. Encouraging a culture of knowledge sharing stimulates innovation and continuous learning. Initiating collaborative projects tackles common issues and improves overall patient care.

Accreditation: Being accredited by a third party is a way for the clinic chain to demonstrate its dedication to quality and safety, which helps it stand out from competitors and gain trust from both patients and staff. This accreditation process involves staff training to improve performance and skills. It also provides a structure for improvement through monitoring and performance evaluation. An important aspect of accreditation is the emphasis on operations to ensure that the clinic chain follows regulations and guidelines, underscoring their commitment to patient care and safety.

16.8 Performance Recognition

Implementing employee recognition programmes that recognise and reward these efforts boosts morale, encourages staff retention, and garners public recognition through avenues like newsletters or social media that can serve as motivation for staff.

Furthermore, actively seeking employee feedback fosters a collaborative environment where employees feel valued and engaged in improvement initiatives. Offering development opportunities related to quality improvement further demonstrates the clinic's commitment to staff growth.

Organising team-building activities that acknowledge the contributions of staff members promotes teamwork, effective communication, and an overall culture of excellence across departments.

Investing in TQMS results in long-term financial benefits for fertility clinics, including reduced costs due to increased efficiency; higher patient satisfaction, leading to increased referrals; and improved employee retention, reducing recruitment and training costs.

CHAPTER 16

SUMMARY

- Safety is paramount in ART labs to protect patients, staff, and the environment.
- Healthcare providers and infertility clinics should prioritise safety by establishing comprehensive safety programmes and regularly reviewing and updating safety protocols.
- Staff should receive proper safety training and follow strict guidelines for handling and disposing of hazardous materials.
- Infertility clinics should have a designated safety officer responsible for overseeing safety measures and maintaining compliance with regulatory standards.
- Fire extinguishers and eye-wash stations, among other emergency supplies, must be easily accessible and always available. Inspections and audits of ART labs identify potential safety hazards and support ongoing safety improvements.
- Training and drills for emergency scenarios prepare staff for unexpected events and improve response times in an emergency.
- ART labs should have proper labelling and identification protocols for hazardous materials to minimise the risk of accidental exposure.

PROPER LABORATORY DESIGN

- It is recommended that laboratories be equipped with appropriate lighting to promote a well-illuminated workspace and minimise the likelihood of mishaps.

- Floors, walls, and ceilings should be constructed of materials that are easy to clean and maintain to minimise the risk of contamination and infection.
- Adequate space should be available to accommodate equipment, staff, and workflow needs.
- Equipment should be properly maintained and regularly calibrated to maintain accuracy and minimise the risk of equipment failure.
- Storage areas for hazardous materials should be adequately ventilated and secure to minimise the risk of accidental exposure or theft.
- Laboratories should have proper signage to identify hazardous materials and emergency equipment.
- Emergency exit routes should be clearly marked, unobstructed, and easily accessible in an emergency.
- Electrical outlets and wiring should be properly grounded and installed to minimise the risk of electrical hazards.
- Laboratories should have proper insulation to maintain a stable temperature and humidity level, which is needed for maintaining the integrity of biological samples.
- The laboratory should be appropriately sealed and have a secure entrance to minimise the risk of unauthorised access.

TQMS FOR A CHAIN OF FERTILITY CLINICS

- Fertility clinic chains have multiple locations and offer a more extensive reach of services, providing convenience and flexibility for patients.
- Advancements in assisted reproductive technologies and increased demand for fertility services have contributed to the growth of fertility clinic chains.
- Fertility clinic chains benefit from resource and expertise pooling; economies of scale; and the ability to provide consistent, high-quality care across multiple locations.
- Implementing a TQMS for a chain of fertility clinics enhances patient care, streamlines operations, and improves overall performance.
- Steps to implement TQMS for a chain of fertility clinics include establishing a clear vision and mission, developing a quality policy, defining key performance indicators, establishing a quality management team, implementing standard operating procedures, utilising technology, fostering a culture of continuous improvement, encouraging collaboration, pursuing accreditation, addressing ethical considerations, and recognising employee performance.

Investing in TQMS results in long-term financial benefits for fertility clinics.

Further Readings

Alikani, M., Cohen, J., Tomkin, G., Garrisi, G. J., Mack, C., & Scott, R. T. (1999). Human embryo fragmentation in vitro and its implications for pregnancy and implantation. *Fertility and Sterility*, *71*(5), 836–842. https://doi.org/10.1016/s0015-0282(99)00092-8. PMID: 10231042.

Alper, M. M., Brinsden, P. R., Fischer, R., & Wikland, M. (2002). Is your IVF programme good? *Human Reproduction*, *17*(1), 8–10. https://doi.org/10.1093/humrep/17.1.8

ASRM Practice Committee. (2008). Revised guidelines for human embryology and andrology laboratories. *Fertility and Sterility*, *90*, S45–S59.

ASRM Practice Committee. (2014). Revised minimum standards for practices offering assisted opinion. *Fertility and Sterility*, *102*, 682–686.

Bento, F., Esteves, S., & Agarwal, A. (2012). *Quality management in ART clinics: A practical guide.* Springer.

Biggers, J. D., & Summers, M. C. (2008). Choosing a culture medium: Making informed choices. *Fertility and Sterility*, *90*(3), 473–483. https://doi.org/10.1016/j.fertnstert.2008.08.010. PMID: 18847602.

Boone, W. R., Johnson, J. E., Locke, A. J., Crane, M. M. IV, & Price, T. M. (1999). Control of air quality in an assisted reproductive technology laboratory. *Fertility and Sterility*, *71*(1), 150–154. https://doi.org/10.1016/s0015-0282(98)00395-1

Cohen, J., Alikani, M., Trowbridge, J., & Rosenwaks, Z. (1992). Implantation enhancement by selective assisted hatching using zona drilling of human embryos with poor prognosis. *Human Reproduction*, *7*(5), 685–691. https://doi.org/10.1093/oxfordjournals.humrep.a137720

Cohen, J., Gilligan, A., Esposito, W., Schimmel, T., & Dale, B. (1997). Ambient air and its potential effects on conception in vitro. *Human Reproduction*, *12*(8), 1742–1749. https://doi.org/10.1093/humrep/12.8.1742. PMID: 9308805.

Cohen, J., Trounson, A., Dawson, K., Jones, H., Hazekamp, J., Nygren, K. G., & Hamberger, L. (2005). The early days of IVF outside the UK. *Human Reproduction Update*, *11*(5), 439–459. https://doi.org/10.1093/humupd/dmi016

Conaghan, J., Chen, A. A., Willman, S. P., Ivani, K., Chenette, P. E., Boostanfar, R., Baker, V. L., Adamson, G. D., Abusief, M. E., Gvakharia, M., Loewke, K. E., & Shen, S. (2013). Improving embryo selection using a computer-automated time-lapse image analysis test plus day 3 morphology: Results from a prospective multicenter trial. *Fertility and Sterility*, *100*(2), 412–419, e5. https://doi.org/10.1016/j.fertnstert.2013.04.021

De Los Santos, M. J., Apter, S., Coticchio, G., Debrock, S., Lundin, K., Plancha, C. E., Prados, F., Rienzi, L., Verheyen, G., Woodward, B., & Vermeulen, N. (2015). Revised guidelines for good practice in IVF laboratories. *Human Reproduction*, *31*, 685–686. http://humrep.oxfordjournals.org/

Dickey, R. P., Pyrzak, R., Lu, P. Y., Taylor, S. N., & Rye, P. H. (1999). Comparison of the sperm quality necessary for successful intrauterine insemination with world health organization threshold values for normal sperm. *Fertility and Sterility*, *71*(4), 684–689. https://doi.org/10.1016/s0015-0282(98)00519-6. PMID: 10202879.

Elder, K., Van Den Bergh, M., & Woodward, B. (2015). *Troubleshooting and problem-solving in the IVF laboratory.* Cambridge University Press.

ESHRE Guideline Group on Good Practice in IVF Labs, De los Santos, M. J., Apter, S., Coticchio, G., Debrock, S., Lundin, K., Plancha, C. E., Prados, F., Rienzi, L., Verheyen, G., Woodward, B., & Vermeulen, N. (2016). Revised guidelines for good practice in IVF laboratories. *Human Reproduction*, *31*(4), 685–686. https://doi.org/10.1093/humrep/dew016. PMID: 26908842.

ESHRE Special Interest Group of Embryology and Alpha Scientists in Reproductive Medicine. (2017). The Vienna consensus: Report of an expert meeting on the development of ART laboratory performance indicators. *Reproductive Biomedicine Online*, *35*, 494–510.

Esteves, S. C., Roque, M., Bedoschi, G., Haahr, T., & Humaidan, P. (2018). Intracytoplasmic sperm injection for male infertility and consequences for offspring. *Nature Reviews Urology*, *15*(9), 535–562. https://doi.org/10.1038/s41585-018-0051-8

Evenson, D. P. (2013). Sperm chromatin structure assay (SCSA®). *Methods in Molecular Biology, 927,* 147–164. https://doi.org/10.1007/978-1-62703-038-0_14. PMID: 22992911.

Fahy, G. M., Wowk, B., & Wu, J. (2006). Cryopreservation of complex systems: The missing link in the regenerative medicine supply chain. *Rejuvenation Research, 9*(2), 279–291. https://doi.org/10.1089/rej.2006.9.279

Ferraretti, A. P., Goossens, V., de Mouzon, J., Bhattacharya, S., Castilla, J. A., Korsak, V., Kupka, M., Nygren, K. G., Nyboe Andersen, A., European IVF-Monitoring (EIM), & Consortium for European Society of Human Reproduction and Embryology (ESHRE). (2012). Assisted reproductive technology in Europe, 2008: Results generated from European registers by ESHRE. *Human Reproduction, 27*(9), 2571–2584. https://doi.org/10.1093/humrep/des255. PMID: 22786779.

Fuller, B. J. (2004). Cryoprotectants: The essential antifreezes to protect life in the frozen state. *Cryo-Letters, 25*(6), 375–388. https://doi.org/10.1080/02535040410002373

Gardner, D. K., & Balaban, B. (2016). Assessment of human embryo development using morphological criteria in an era of time-lapse, algorithms and "OMICS": Is looking good still important? *Molecular Human Reproduction, 22*(10), 704–718. https://doi.org/10.1093/molehr/gaw057

Gardner, D. K., Meseguer, M., Rubio, C., & Treff, N. R. (2015). Diagnosis of human preimplantation embryo viability. *Human Reproduction Update, 21*(6), 727–747. https://doi.org/10.1093/humupd/dmu064

Gianaroli, L., Plachot, M., van Kooij, R., Al-Hasani, S., Dawson, K., DeVos, A., Magli, M. C., Mandelbaum, J., Selva, J., & van Inzen, W. (2000). ESHRE guidelines for good practice in IVF laboratories: Committee of the special interest group on embryology of the European society of human reproduction and embryology. *Human Reproduction, 10,* 2241–2246.

Gook, D. A., & Edgar, D. H. (2007). Human oocyte cryopreservation. *Human Reproduction Update, 13*(6), 591–605. https://doi.org/10.1093/humupd/dmm028

Haidl, G., Badura, B., Hinsch, K. D., Ghyczy, M., Gareiss, J., & Schill, W. B. (1993). Disturbances of sperm flagella due to failure of epididymal maturation and their possible relationship to phospholipids. *Human Reproduction, 8*(7), 1070–1073. https://doi.org/10.1093/oxfordjournals.humrep.a138194. PMID: 8408489.

Hardarson, T., Bungum, M., Conaghan, J., Meintjes, M., Chantilis, S. J., Molnar, L., Gunnarsson, K., & Wikland, M. (2015). Noninferiority, randomized, controlled trial comparing embryo development using media developed for sequential or undisturbed culture in a time-lapse setup. *Fertility and Sterility, 104*(6), 1452–1459, e1–e4. https://doi.org/10.1016/j.fertnstert.2015.08.037. PMID: 26409153.

Harper, J., Jackson, E., Sermon, K., Aitken, R. J., Harbottle, S., Mocanu, E., Hardarson, T., Mathur, R., Viville, S., Vail, A., & Lundin, K. (2017). Adjuncts in the IVF laboratory: Where is the evidence for "add-on" interventions? *Human Reproduction, 32*(3), 485–491. https://doi.org/10.1093/humrep/dex004. PMID: 28158511.

Harper, J., Magli, M. C., Lundin, K., Barratt, C. L., & Brison, D. (2012). When and how should new technology be introduced into the IVF laboratory? *Human Reproduction, 27*(2), 303–313. https://doi.org/10.1093/humrep/der414

Henkel, R. R., & Schill, W. B. (2003). Sperm preparation for ART. *Reproductive Biology and Endocrinology, 1,* 108. https://doi.org/10.1186/1477-7827-1-108. PMID: 14617368; PMCID: PMC293422.

Houghton, F. D. (2005). Role of gap junctions during early embryo development. *Reproduction, 129*(2), 129–135. https://doi.org/10.1530/rep.1.00277. PMID: 15695607.

Huggett, J. F., Foy, C. A., Benes, V., Emslie, K., Garson, J. A., Haynes, R., Hellemans, J., Kubista, M., Mueller, R. D., Nolan, T., Pfaffl, M. W., Shipley, G. L., Vandesompele, J., Wittwer, C. T., & Bustin, S. A. (2013). The digital MIQE guidelines: Minimum information for publication of quantitative digital PCR experiments. *Clinical Chemistry, 59*(6), 892–902. https://doi.org/10.1373/clinchem.2013.206375. PMID: 23570709.

Khoudja, R. Y., Xu, Y., Li, T., & Zhou, C. (2013). Better IVF outcomes following improvements in laboratory air quality. *Journal of Assisted Reproduction and Genetics, 30*(1), 69–76. https://doi.org/10.1007/s10815-012-9900-1. PMID: 23242648; PMCID: PMC3553352.

Lane, M., & Gardner, D. K. (2007). Embryo culture medium: Which is the best? *Best Practice & Research Clinical Obstetrics & Gynaecology, 21*(1), 83–100. https://doi.org/10.1016/j.bpobgyn.2006.09.009. PMID: 17090393.

Lucena, E., Bernal, D. P., Lucena, C., Rojas, A., Moran, A., & Lucena, A. (2006). Successful ongoing pregnancies after vitrification of oocytes. *Fertility and Sterility*, *85*(1), 108–111. https://doi.org/10.1016/j.fertnstert.2005.09.013. PMID: 16412739.

Magli, C., Van den Abbeel, E., Lundin, K., Royere, D., Van der Elst, J., & Gianaroli, L. (2008). Revised guidelines for good practice in IVF laboratories. *Human Reproduction*, *23*, 1253–1260.

Mains, L., & Van Voorhis, B. J. (2010). Optimizing the technique of embryo transfer. *Fertility and Sterility*, *94*(3), 785–790. https://doi.org/10.1016/j.fertnstert.2010.03.030. PMID: 20409543.

Malhotra, N., Shah, D., Pai, R., Pai, H. D., & Bankar, M. (2013). Assisted reproductive technology in India: A 3 year retrospective data analysis. *Journal of Human Reproductive Sciences*, *6*(4), 235.

Meseguer, M., Rubio, I., Cruz, M., Basile, N., Marcos, J., & Requena, A. (2012). Embryo incubation and selection in a time-lapse monitoring system improves pregnancy outcome compared with a standard incubator: A retrospective cohort study. *Fertility and Sterility*, *98*(6), 1481–1489, e10. https://doi.org/10.1016/j.fertnstert.2012.08.016. PMID: 22975113.

Montgomery, D. C. (2020). *Introduction to statistical quality control* (8th ed.). Wiley.

Morbeck, D. E., Krisher, R. L., Herrick, J. R., Baumann, N. A., Matern, D., & Moyer, T. (2014). Composition of commercial media used for human embryo culture. *Fertility and Sterility*, *102*(3), 759–766, e9. https://doi.org/10.1016/j.fertnstert.2014.05.043. PMID: 24998366.

Morbeck, D. E., Paczkowski, M., Fredrickson, J. R., Krisher, R. L., Hoff, H. S., Baumann, N. A., Moyer, T., & Matern, D. (2014). Composition of protein supplements used for human embryo culture. *Journal of Assisted Reproduction and Genetics*, *31*(12), 1703–1711. https://doi.org/10.1007/s10815-014-0349-2. PMID: 25261352; PMCID: PMC4250459.

Mortimer, D., Cohen, J., Mortimer, S. T., Fawzy, M., McCulloh, D. H., Morbeck, D. E., Pollet-Villard, X., Mansour, R. T., Brison, D. R., Doshi, A., Harper, J. C., Swain, J. E., & Gilligan, A. V. (2018). Cairo consensus on the IVF laboratory environment and air quality: Report of an expert meeting. *Reproductive Biomedicine Online*, *36*(6), 658–674. https://doi.org/10.1016/j.rbmo.2018.02.005. PMID: 29656830.

Mortimer, D., & Mortimer, S. T. (2005). *Quality and risk management in the IVF laboratory*. Cambridge University Press.

Palermo, G. D., Neri, Q. V., Cozzubbo, T., & Rosenwaks, Z. (2014). Perspectives on the assessment of human sperm chromatin integrity. *Fertility and Sterility*, *102*(6), 1508–1517. https://doi.org/10.1016/j.fertnstert.2014.10.008

Petersen, P. H., Stöckl, D., Blaabjerg, O., Pedersen, B., Birkemose, E., Thienpont, L., Lassen, J. F., & Kjeldsen, J. (1997). Graphical interpretation of analytical data from comparison of a field method with a reference method by use of difference plots. *Clinical Chemistry*, *43*(11), 2039–2046. PMID: 9365386.

Pool, T. B. (2005). An update on embryo culture for human assisted reproductive technology: Media, performance, and safety. *Seminars in Reproductive Medicine*, *23*(4), 309–318. https://doi.org/10.1055/s-2005-923388. PMID: 16317619.

Pool, T. B., Schoolfield, J., & Han, D. K. (2012). Human embryo culture media practice committee of the American society for reproductive medicine and the practice committee of the society for assisted reproductive technology, 2013. Recommendations for gamete and embryo donation: A committee opinion. *Fertility and Sterility*, *99*(1), 47–62, e1. https://doi.org/10.1016/j.fertnstert.2012.09.037

Pool, T. B., Schoolfield, J., & Han, D. (2012). Human embryo culture media comparisons. *Embryo Culture: Methods and Protocols*, 367–386. https://doi.org/10.1007/978-1-61779-971-6_21

Racowsky, C., Vernon, M., Mayer, J., Ball, G. D., Behr, B., Pomeroy, K. O., Wininger, D., Gibbons, W., Conaghan, J., & Stern, J. E. (2010). Standardization of grading embryo morphology. *Fertility and Sterility*, *94*(3), 1152–1153. https://doi.org/10.1016/j.fertnstert.2010.05.042. PMID: 20580357.

Rienzi, L., Bariani, F., Dalla Zorza, M., Albani, E., Benini, F., Chamayou, S., Minasi, M. G., Parmegiani, L., Restelli, L., Vizziello, G., & Costa, A. N. (2017). Comprehensive protocol of traceability during IVF: The result of a multicentre failure mode and effect analysis. *Human Reproduction*, *32*(8), 1612–1620. https://doi.org/10.1093/humrep/dex144

Rienzi, L., Bariani, F., Dalla Zorza, M., Romano, S., Scarica, C., Maggiulli, R., Nanni Costa, A., & Ubaldi, F. M. (2015). Failure mode and effects analysis of witnessing protocols for ensuring traceability during IVF. *Reproductive Biomedicine Online*, *31*(4), 516–522. https://doi.org/10.1016/j.rbmo.2015.06.018

Rienzi, L., Gracia, C., Maggiulli, R., LaBarbera, A. R., Kaser, D. J., Ubaldi, F. M., Vanderpoel, S., & Racowsky, C. (2017). Oocyte, embryo and blastocyst cryopreservation in ART: Systematic review and meta-analysis comparing slow-freezing versus vitrification to produce evidence for the development of global guidance. *Human Reproduction Update*, 23(2), 139–155. https://doi.org/10.1093/humupd/dmw038. PMID: 27827818; PMCID: PMC5850862.

Rienzi, L., Ubaldi, F., Anniballo, R., Cerulo, G., & Greco, E. (1998). Preincubation of human oocytes may improve fertilization and embryo quality after intracytoplasmic sperm injection. *Human Reproduction*, 13(4), 1014–1019. https://doi.org/10.1093/humrep/13.4.1014. PMID: 9619563.

Sakkas, D., Ramalingam, M., Garrido, N., & Barratt, C. L. (2015). Sperm selection in natural conception: What can we learn from Mother Nature to improve assisted reproduction outcomes? *Human Reproduction Update*, 21(6), 711–726. https://doi.org/10.1093/humupd/dmv042. PMID: 26386468; PMCID: PMC4594619.

Salamonsen, L. A., Evans, J., Nguyen, H. P., & Edgell, T. A. (2016). The microenvironment of human implantation: Determinant of reproductive success. *American Journal of Reproductive Immunology*, 75(3), 218–225. https://doi.org/10.1111/aji.12450

Sharma, R., Biedenharn, K. R., Fedor, J. M., & Agarwal, A. (2013). Lifestyle factors and reproductive health: Taking control of your fertility. *Reproductive Biology and Endocrinology*, 11, 66. https://doi.org/10.1186/1477-7827-11-66. PMID: 23870423; PMCID: PMC3717046.

Shenfield, F., de Mouzon, J., Pennings, G., Ferraretti, A. P., Andersen, A. N., de Wert, G., Goossens, V., & ESHRE Taskforce on Cross Border Reproductive Care. (2010). Cross border reproductive care in six European countries. *Human Reproduction*, 25(6), 1361–1368. https://doi.org/10.1093/humrep/deq057. PMID: 20348165.

Simón, C., Escobedo, C., Valbuena, D., Genbacev, O., Galan, A., Krtolica, A., Asensi, A., Sánchez, E., Esplugues, J., Fisher, S., & Pellicer, A. (2005). First derivation in Spain of human embryonic stem cell lines: Use of long-term cryopreserved embryos and animal-free conditions. *Fertility and Sterility*, 83(1), 246–249. https://doi.org/10.1016/j.fertnstert.2004.09.004. PMID: 15652923.

Souter, I., Baltagi, L. M., Kuleta, D., Meeker, J. D., & Petrozza, J. C. (2011). Women, weight, and fertility: The effect of body mass index on the outcome of superovulation/intrauterine insemination cycles. *Fertility and Sterility*, 95(3), 1042–1047. https://doi.org/10.1016/j.fertnstert.2010.11.062. PMID: 21195401.

Swain, J. E. (2014). Decisions for the IVF laboratory: Comparative analysis of embryo culture incubators. *Reproductive Biomedicine Online*, 28(5), 535–547. https://doi.org/10.1016/j.rbmo.2014.01.004. PMID: 24656561.

Talbot, P., & Riveles, K. (2005). Smoking and reproduction: The oviduct as a target of cigarette smoke. *Reproductive Biology and Endocrinology*, 3, 52. https://doi.org/10.1186/1477-7827-3-52. PMID: 16191196; PMCID: PMC1266059.

Tarlatzis, B. C., Zepiridis, L., Grimbizis, G., & Bontis, J. (2003). Clinical management of low ovarian response to stimulation for IVF: A systematic review. *Human Reproduction Update*, 9(1), 61–76. https://doi.org/10.1093/humupd/dmg007

Vajta, G., & Nagy, Z. P. (2006). Are programmable freezers still needed in the embryo laboratory? Review on vitrification. *Reproductive Biomedicine Online*, 12(6), 779–796. https://doi.org/10.1016/s1472-6483(10)61091-7. PMID: 16792858.

Varghese, A. C., Sjoblom, P., & Jayaprakasan, K. (2013). *A practical guide to setting up an IVF lab, embryo culture systems and running the unit.* Jaypee Brothers Medical Publishers (P) Ltd.

Yao, N., Yang, X. F., Zhu, B., Liao, C. Y., He, Y. M., Du, J., Liu, N., & Zhou, C. B. (2022). Bacterial colonization on healthcare workers' mobile phones and hands in municipal hospitals of Chongqing, China: Cross-contamination and associated factors. *Journal of Epidemiology and Global Health*, 12, 390–399. https://doi.org/10.1007/s44197-022-00057-1

Zegers-Hochschild, F., Adamson, G. D., de Mouzon, J., Ishihara, O., Mansour, R., Nygren, K., Sullivan, E., Vanderpoel, S., International Committee for Monitoring Assisted Reproductive Technology, & World Health Organization. (2009). International committee for monitoring assisted reproductive technology (ICMART) and the world health organization (WHO) revised glossary of ART terminology, 2009. *Fertility and Sterility*, 92(5), 1520–1524. https://doi.org/10.1016/j.fertnstert.2009.09.009. PMID: 19828144.

Zegers-Hochschild, F., Adamson, G. D., Dyer, S., Racowsky, C., de Mouzon, J., Sokol, R., Rienzi, L., Sunde, A., Schmidt, L., Cooke, I. D., Simpson, J. L., & van der Poel, S. (2017). The international glossary on infertility and fertility care, 2017. *Fertility and Sterility*, *108*(3), 393–406. https://doi.org/10.1016/j.fertnstert.2017.06.005. PMID: 28760517.

Zegers-Hochschild, F., Adamson, G. D., Dyer, S., Racowsky, C., de Mouzon, J., Sokol, R., Rienzi, L., Sunde, A., Schmidt, L., Cooke, I. D., Simpson, J. L., & van der Poel, S. (2017). The international glossary on infertility and fertility care, 2017. *Human Reproduction*, *32*(9), 1786–1801. https://doi.org/10.1093/humrep/dex234

Index

Note: Page numbers in *italics* indicate a figure and page numbers in **bold** indicate a table on the corresponding page.